The Runner's Guide to Menopause

Dr Juliet McGrattan

The Runner's Guide to Menopause

Your essential toolkit for strong, happy and healthy training

Dr Juliet McGrattan

BLOOMSBURY SPORT
LONDON · OXFORD · NEW YORK · NEW DELHI · SYDNEY

BLOOMSBURY SPORT
Bloomsbury Publishing Plc
50 Bedford Square, London, WC1B 3DP, UK
Bloomsbury Publishing Ireland Limited
29 Earlsfort Terrace, Dublin 2, D02 AY28, Ireland

BLOOMSBURY, BLOOMSBURY SPORT and the Diana logo are trademarks
of Bloomsbury Publishing Plc

First published in Great Britain 2026

Copyright © Juliet McGrattan, 2026
Additional text, training plans and exercises by Clare Clark, Irene Clark and Renee McGregor

Juliet McGrattan has asserted her right under the Copyright, Designs and Patents Act, 1988,
to be identified as Author of this work

For legal purposes the Acknowledgements on p. 311
constitute an extension of this copyright page

All rights reserved. No part of this publication may be: i) reproduced or transmitted in any form, electronic or mechanical, including photocopying, recording or by means of any information storage or retrieval system without prior permission in writing from the publishers; or ii) used or reproduced in any way for the training, development or operation of artificial intelligence (AI) technologies, including generative AI technologies. The rights holders expressly reserve this publication from the text and data mining exception as per Article 4(3) of the Digital Single Market Directive (EU) 2019/790

Bloomsbury Publishing Plc does not have any control over, or responsibility for, any third-party websites referred to or in this book. All internet addresses given in this book were correct at the time of going to press. The author and publisher regret any inconvenience caused if addresses have changed or sites have ceased to exist, but can accept no responsibility for any such changes

The information contained in this book is provided by way of general guidance in relation to the specific subject matters addressed herein, but it is not a substitute for specialist advice. It should not be relied on for medical, health-care, pharmaceutical or other professional advice on specific dietary or health needs. This book is sold with the understanding that the author and publisher are not engaged in rendering medical, health or any other kind of personal or professional services. The reader should consult a competent medical or health professional before adopting any of the suggestions in this book or drawing inferences from it. The author and publisher specifically disclaim, as far as the law allows, any responsibility from any liability, loss or risk (personal or otherwise) which is incurred as a consequence, directly or indirectly, of the use and applications of any of the contents of this book.

A catalogue record for this book is available from the British Library

Library of Congress Cataloguing-in-Publication data has been applied for

ISBN: TPB: 978-1-3994-2385-4; eBook: 978-1-3994-2388-5

2 4 6 8 10 9 7 5 3 1

Typeset in Source Serif Pro by Lumina Datamatics Ltd
Printed and bound in Great Britain by Clays Ltd, Elcograf S.p.A.

To find out more about our authors and books visit www.bloomsbury.com
and sign up for our newsletters
For product safety related questions contact productsafety@bloomsbury.com

Contents

Preface *vii*

Introduction *1*

CHAPTER 1 **What is Menopause?** *4*

CHAPTER 2 **Benefits and Challenges** *13*

CHAPTER 3 **Flushes and Sweats** *19*

CHAPTER 4 **Sleep** *28*

CHAPTER 5 **Energy Levels** *37*

CHAPTER 6 **Periods** *49*

CHAPTER 7 **Breasts** *58*

CHAPTER 8 **Bladders and Bits** *68*

CHAPTER 9 **Bowels** *79*

CHAPTER 10 **Bones and Joints** *90*

CHAPTER 11 **Muscles and Tendons** *105*

CHAPTER 12 **Body Composition** *120*

CHAPTER 13 **Skin** *132*

CHAPTER 14 **Mental Health** *143*

CHAPTER 15 **Menopause Treatments** *157*

CHAPTER 16 **Nutrition** *178*

CHAPTER 17 **Training** *198*

CHAPTER 18 **Training Plans** *213*

CHAPTER 19 **Strength** *270*

CHAPTER 20 **Mindset** *302*

Closing Words *310*

Acknowledgements *311*

References *312*

Index *324*

Preface

I began running aged 35. I'm now 53 and I have many miles and marathons under my belt, but I vividly recall the first time perimenopause interfered with my running. I was taking my usual route along the country lanes surrounding my village. I began struggling up a hill I could usually run with ease. I was so out of breath, the colour of a tomato and sweating excessively. Perimenopause has continued to affect my running in a variety of ways from that day on. I've been upset, frustrated, at times run less and even wondered whether I could still call myself a runner.

I worked as a GP for 16 years and during that time I saw hundreds of women at different stages of menopause. I witnessed the huge impact it had on all areas of their lives, but it wasn't until I hit perimenopause myself that I truly understood how it feels. I began to realise that every bit of my body was changing and that had a negative knock-on effect on my running, both in terms of how well I could run, but also in terms of how I felt about running. I wasn't expecting this and I didn't like it!

I've spent the last decade helping women into running, through writing about the barriers to running, by working with 261 Fearless, a global, social running network which creates opportunities for women around the world to run, and by literally taking women by the hand as a running coach. I'm passionate about the power of running for women and I've witnessed it change lives. Women generally become less active when menopause hits, yet it's a time when we need the power of running more than ever. Our disease risk is increasing, our muscles and bones are weakening, and we can feel lost and vulnerable. The consequences of running less negatively affect our physical, mental and social health. Our health in old age is hugely influenced by what we do now. It's unfair that for most women, the barriers to being active get higher in menopause.

Let's be honest, life is better with running in it. Running can make us feel successful, strong and fit. It grows our self-confidence, self-belief and makes us feel alive. It brings fun, friends and a connection with others and with nature. It also helps us to cope with change and to navigate uncertainty and turbulent times. For all these reasons, we need running to help us manage this life transition and set us up for a healthy future.

Alongside my own experiences, lots of you started telling me just how hard you were finding it to keep running in menopause and this spurred me into action. My next challenge was clear: researching and writing a book to help women to keep running during menopause and beyond. And, several years later, here it is. A book for all of you: for the ultramarathon runners among you to the very occasional parkrunner; for the women who inspire me, the women who run alongside me and the women I have yet to meet. Whether you have run all your life or have just begun a Couch to 5km, this is for you. Written from the heart and the science, with my straight-talking, sensible and realistic approach, I sincerely hope it helps you to keep running through menopause and enjoy strong, happy and healthy training.

Introduction

Every woman's experience of menopause is different. For some, symptoms are minimal, and life and running isn't disrupted much at all. For others, just getting through each day is a real challenge and running can feel out of the question. Wherever you are on this spectrum, I hope you will find tips, information and inspiration in this book. We'll be going from hot flushes in chapter 3 to frozen shoulders in chapter 11; from shrinking breasts in chapter 7 to expanding waistlines in chapter 12. We'll find fixes, share stories and quash some menopause myths along the way.

But we're not stopping there. If you're feeling overwhelmed by the confusing nutritional information on your social media feeds, then head to chapter 16 to find out what you should put in your shopping basket. If your running just isn't going well or you know you want to start some strength work, then dive into chapters 17, 18 and 19 for expert training advice, from lifting your first weight through to an advanced marathon training plan. Our target is sustainable and healthy training, but please remember that this book is general guidance and it doesn't replace seeing a healthcare professional who can give you personalised advice and treatment.

From the outset, I want to acknowledge that menopause evokes different emotions and feelings in all of us. It marks the end of our reproductive years. For some women this brings relief and liberation, for others it can bring sadness and grief. This can particularly be the case in women who have an early or premature menopause. Our attitude to menopause can also be determined by our cultural norms. The topic is still taboo, particularly in minority communities. Many women are expected to just get on with menopause without complaint. It can even be seen as a loss of femininity. In some African cultures, however, ageing women are valued and called 'Queen' as a sign of respect.

There are around one billion people around the world in peri- or post-menopause, and this includes women, trans-masculine, non-binary and intersex people. I'm using the term woman throughout this book to include anyone who was assigned female at birth, but we're all different, and it's vital we acknowledge this and are all part of the conversation. Let's be open to learning from each other, and curious and respectful of our different approaches and experiences.

I'm not going to pretend that running in menopause is easy. This is a huge time of change for our bodies, and it often results in increased barriers to running and reduced performance. We need to be proactive, adapt and make changes if we want to continue to get the best out of our running. I firmly believe that movement is a very powerful medicine and every action we take to be able to keep active is most definitely worth it. We have hard work ahead of us, but the rewards are enormous.

I'm also not going to pretend that I have all the answers. Research on women and menopause has a lot of catching up to do. It can be hard to distinguish what is due to menopause and what is due to ageing. Don't be swayed by new fads, trends and influencers with magic solutions. There is so much we don't know and one size will never fit all. The contents of this book are my take on running and menopause based on current, credible evidence, but at the end of the day doing what feels right for you, and allows you to exercise in an enjoyable and consistent way, is always best.

It's easy to undervalue what running does for you. You might think your running isn't serious enough to be relevant and it wouldn't really matter if you didn't do it at all. I want you to know that it absolutely does matter; it matters just as much to you as it does to the most serious of runners. It's vitally important for your present and future physical, mental and social health.

If you seem to have fallen out of love with running, take a moment to think back to when you started and first discovered its magic and power. What did it bring you? Calmness, strength and belief in yourself? Fun, resilience and happiness? The very things it gave you then are the benefits you need now. Some days, when running is hard and you feel like a beginner again, it can get you down, but perhaps you could use it as an opportunity to relish the rediscovery of running. Make space for it to grow your confidence, calm your anxiety and turn bad days into good, just as it did for you before. Running is a wonderful gift to help us in menopause, even if it looks and feels different.

A healthy lifestyle is the number one prescription when it comes to menopause, but if you're in the thick of it, finding the extra effort and enthusiasm to address that can feel overwhelming. Where do you even begin? Changing your behaviour and creating new habits and routines is difficult, but there are two pieces of good news. Firstly, research has proven that transition times in life, such as getting a new job, a child leaving for university or being diagnosed with a medical condition, are the best times to make a change. They are an opportunity for a complete reset. Menopause is one such transition. Secondly, you don't have to do it all at once. You don't need one massive life overhaul, because trying to change too much in one go can stop you starting or being able to sustain it. Instead, look for an easy win. Change that and do it over and over again, until it becomes a habit, and then move on to a new, tiny thing. Small changes really do add up and even if the positive step you make today feels like nothing, it can have a huge impact in the long term. Taking a 10-minute walk before you start work or standing up whenever you're making a phone call might seem insignificant and not worth doing, but if you do them every day, over time they'll significantly increase your activity levels and have an impact on your future health.

There is a societal expectation that we will do less as we age; that we've reached our peak, become fragile and it's all downhill from here. Women are led to believe that their demise begins at the time of menopause. We'll spend around one-third to one-half of our lives in post-menopause. I, for one, am not prepared to accept that half my life will be inferior to the rest. Thankfully, there are many post-menopausal women out there showing us that decline is not inevitable, because they are thriving in life and running. They are proof that there is a bright, shining light at the end of the menopause tunnel. There is hope, plenty of it. On some days it can feel like the beginning of the end, but it's important to remember that what is happening to us is not our fault, it is our hormones and this phase of our lives doesn't last forever, it is transient.

We're at a point where we can make a decision. We can choose to let our running slide or we can embrace the often ugly, exhilarating rollercoaster of running in menopause and come off it knowing that despite the loop-the-loops, the feelings of loss of control and the occasional nausea, we hung on, are proud of ourselves and, dare I say it, enjoyed the ride. While managing menopause is not always easy, running is a wonderful tool to help you. I don't want you to fall out of love with running or lose the joy that running has brought you. I want you to reap all the health benefits that running has to offer and I hope this book helps you to keep going.

CHAPTER 1

What is Menopause?

The more we understand what menopause actually is and what's going on in our bodies, the easier it is to see why we feel the way we do. This will help us identify the solutions.

THE MENSTRUAL CYCLE

First, let's recap the basics of hormones and the menstrual cycle. Menarche is what we officially call the start of menstrual periods. The average age this happens in the UK is 13. Periods can be erratic initially, but after a year or so they've usually settled into a regular pattern. The cycle starts on day one when period bleeding begins. Stimulated by a rise in follicle-stimulating hormone (FSH), oestrogen levels increase and an ovarian follicle develops and prepares to release an egg. Ovulation (egg release) usually happens around day 14 and is triggered by a surge in luteinising hormone (LH). After ovulation, progesterone levels rise and the body prepares for a potential pregnancy. If there's no pregnancy, then oestrogen and progesterone levels fall and bleeding starts, bringing us back round to the beginning of the cycle again. The whole cycle can take anywhere from 20 to 40 days.

The hypothalamus in the brain monitors the levels of circulating oestrogen and progesterone in the blood, and messages the pituitary gland, also in the brain, via a hormone called gonadotropin-releasing hormone (GnRH), to tell it whether it needs more or less oestrogen and progesterone. The pituitary gland makes FSH and LH, and according to the instructions from the hypothalamus, it releases larger or smaller amounts of these hormones into the bloodstream. When they reach the ovaries, they determine the production of oestrogen and progesterone. This whole system is called the hypothalamic-pituitary-ovarian axis and it controls the reproductive cycle.

WHAT HAPPENS IN MENOPAUSE?

When ovarian function declines and egg numbers are low, the amount of oestrogen and progesterone produced in the ovaries decreases. FSH levels will rise to try to stimulate more oestrogen and LH levels will increase to attempt to induce ovulation. Ovulation doesn't always happen and a cycle without ovulation is called an anovulatory cycle. These types of cycle are common just after menarche and before menopause, and they're typically irregular, with differing amounts of bleeding. Eventually, periods stop altogether and when you haven't had one for 12 months, you reach menopause. The ovaries can still make a little bit of oestrogen, but levels in the body are around 10 per cent of what they were before menopause. Oestrogen isn't just made in the ovaries, it's also made in fat cells and the adrenal glands, which are located just above each kidney, and there are different types:

- Oestradiol (E2) – produced in the ovaries and the main player during our reproductive years.
- Oestrone (E1) – made in the adrenals and fatty tissue, and our main oestrogen after menopause.
- Oestriol (E3) – made by the placenta and the primary oestrogen during pregnancy.

Testosterone reduces slowly from around age 35 and there is no sudden drop in menopause. After menopause the ovaries are still able to make about half of the body's testosterone requirements; the rest is made in the adrenal glands.

> ## GOOD TO KNOW
> You're born with one to two million follicles in your ovaries, each containing an egg. There are around 300,000 to 500,000 left once you start puberty. Even though one follicle releases its egg each menstrual cycle, you lose around 1000 follicles each month and at menopause there are generally around 1000 left.

THE TIMING OF MENOPAUSE

Menopause is actually a single day: the day you haven't had a period for 12 consecutive months. Any time before that is called pre-menopause and any time after is post-menopause. The time leading up to the day of menopause, when symptoms related to hormone changes begin, is called the perimenopause. Lots of factors determine the age at which you reach menopause. The average age in the UK is 51, but any age after 45 is considered normal. Ethnicity is very important here. For example, Indian women tend to have their menopause an average of five years earlier than white women. For women of African-Caribbean descent, menopause is usually one to two years earlier with an average age of 49.6. Other medical conditions can have an influence, too. Women with polycystic ovary syndrome (PCOS) can reach menopause around two years later than those without the condition. Globally, women from low-income countries tend to have an earlier menopause than those from high-income countries. The age at which your periods start (menarche) doesn't always determine when you will reach menopause, but if your menarche is delayed beyond the age of 16 or 17, you may reach menopause a year or so later than someone who had their menarche aged 13.

If you're between 40 and 45 when you reach menopause it's called an early menopause. This happens to at least 12 per cent of women. If you're less than 40, it's classed as a premature menopause, often caused by premature ovarian insufficiency (POI). Premature menopause affects around 4 per cent of women, some of whom are girls, as this can happen at any age.

> 'I went through ovarian failure [POI] in my early thirties and found it very difficult to speak to anyone about the impact it had on me and what it meant for my health. Only recently, 15 years later, have I had the courage to ask for help.'
>
> **Alice Penn,** London

Menopause happens for a variety of reasons. The most common is a natural menopause determined by the internal programming of your body. There is a genetic element here, although it's not fully understood. POI can sometimes run in families. Menopause can also be induced and sudden. For example, if you have surgery that removes your ovaries, it's called a surgically induced menopause. Interestingly, this can also happen when just the uterus is removed (hysterectomy) and the ovaries remain, but the process can still trigger menopause. A medically induced menopause can occur as a result of treatments such as chemotherapy or radiotherapy, or with certain medical conditions such as autoimmune diseases or after a mumps infection.

MENOPAUSE TERMINOLOGY

In this book, when I use the terms menopause and menopausal I mean women who are perimenopausal, but also women who are in the first few years after menopause, when they are still very likely to have the symptoms and their bodies haven't fully adjusted to post-menopausal life. Post-menopausal women tell me they often feel excluded when everything they read is directed towards perimenopausal women. Sadly, there isn't a magic switch that turns off all menopause symptoms when that day of menopause is reached. The average number of years women are affected is seven, but one in three women experience symptoms for longer than that, even up to 10 years or more, and, despite being classed as post-menopausal, women tell me they still feel very much menopausal. The information and advice in this book is useful for post-menopausal women too.

> 'I'm still perimenopausal. My record stretch without a period is 211 days. It's become a family joke that whenever I get a period the count goes back to zero.'
>
> **Anonymous,** age 52

THE MENOPAUSE EXPERIENCE

The production of ovarian hormones doesn't decline in a nice, steady, gradual way in perimenopause, it oscillates up and down and it's the fluctuations in the hormone levels that cause the majority of symptoms. There are oestrogen receptors in a wide variety of tissues and organs, so the extent of symptoms is vast and covers every system in the body, either directly or indirectly.

Some women experience very few menopause symptoms and others tick off everything on the list. You might be mildly affected, but your friend is debilitated. The British Menopause Society reports that menopause symptoms affect over 75 per cent of women and 25 per cent of those women describe their symptoms as severe. However, we shouldn't forget that there are women who don't have symptoms or have very mild ones that don't interfere with their lives. The picture painted is very much one of doom and gloom, but there are women who go through menopause with very little disruption.

GOOD TO KNOW

In the media, menopausal women are often older women, looking sweaty and holding a fan. This is an inaccurate and unhelpful representation of women in menopause. Most women will experience menopause symptoms in their forties and even younger if they have POI. We need to change the narrative, talk about menopause more and make everyone aware of the symptoms and when they can begin. Menopause is not just about old women!

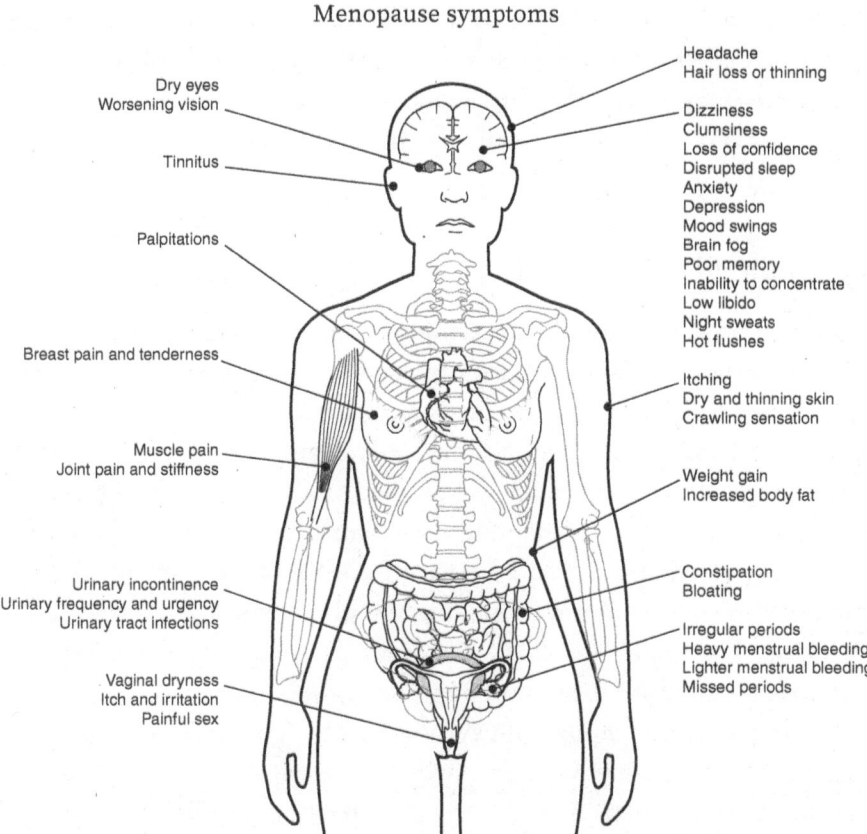

DIAGNOSING MENOPAUSE

Knowing if you're perimenopausal or if you've reached menopause isn't always straightforward. The most important clue indicating perimenopause is the onset of symptoms. In the UK, the average age when these start is 47. The first symptom, in early perimenopause, is usually a change in your menstrual cycle. However, there are many women who begin with other symptoms first, such as hot flushes, fatigue or feelings of anxiety. This is where it gets tricky, because of course, these symptoms can be caused by so many other things. Perimenopause may not be the first thing that springs to your mind or even to your doctor's as the root cause of your issues. Feelings of anxiety might be attributed to work or family stress rather than to changing hormones, so education is crucial.

The more we know, the more confident we can feel about trusting our bodies and advocating for ourselves. Thankfully, there has been a push to educate health professionals about menopause, and awareness and knowledge is increasing all the time.

Do you need a blood test?

You might have seen menopause blood tests being advertised privately or felt disgruntled if your doctor didn't offer to test you, but there isn't a blood test that will tell you exactly where you are on the menopause spectrum. Don't waste your money. The levels of hormones during perimenopause are up, down and all over the place. A blood test only gives you a snapshot in time and that's not helpful. You could have a completely normal test and be right in the throes of perimenopause. The most important thing in making the diagnosis is your symptoms. Checking hormonal levels is not recommended or necessary to diagnose menopause in women over the age of 45.

There are a few important caveats. Firstly, if you are under 45 and would be classed as having an early or premature menopause, then you need a diagnosis based on your hormonal profiles, because, if menopause is confirmed, you may need or want treatment (see chapter 15). Two blood tests, four to six weeks apart, measuring FSH are required. FSH will be very high, as the pituitary will be sending out lots of it to try and stimulate oestrogen production in the ovaries.

> ### GOOD TO KNOW
> Using hormonal contraception doesn't postpone your menopause. It might mask some of the symptoms of perimenopause, but it won't delay the time at which your menopause begins or ends.

If you're using progestogen-only contraception that stops your periods, such as an intrauterine system (IUS) or progestogen injection, you may have no idea whether your menstrual cycle has changed, because you don't have one! It's impossible to know exactly when you've reached that day of menopause. You might realise you're perimenopausal from other symptoms, but you won't know when you move into post-menopause. That doesn't necessarily matter, but there might be situations where you want to know your menopause status, for example if you'd like to stop progestogen-only contraception. Combined hormonal contraceptives and HRT both suppress hormone levels, so you won't get accurate information about your menopausal status from a blood test if you're using these either.

The other situation when you might need to have blood tests is if your doctor wants to rule out other conditions. For example, they might want to make sure your fatigue isn't caused by an underactive thyroid or anaemia (see chapter 5).

> 'I had palpitations, brain fog and difficulty speaking sometimes. My sister had had thyroid cancer, so I wanted to have blood tests to rule out any medical problems. I had a very good, understanding GP, who listened.'
> **Nikki Carpenter**

GOOD TO KNOW

Avoid over-the-counter or internet menopause testing kits using saliva or urine, because they aren't a reliable indicator of whether you are in perimenopause and can even be misleading. They are not recommended by the British Menopause Society nor found in any guidelines for menopause treatment. If someone is suggesting these tests to you either for diagnosis or monitoring of menopause, then check their medical credentials.

When should I go to the doctor?

You don't necessarily need to see the doctor to confirm you are perimenopausal. The diagnosis can be made on symptoms alone if you are over 45 years of age. However, you should go and see a doctor or practice nurse if:

- You think you are in perimenopause and you are under 45 years of age.
- You aren't certain that your symptoms are due to perimenopause.
- Your symptoms are affecting your daily life.
- You have other medical or health concerns that you think might be affected by menopause.

For more about symptoms and when to see your doctor, see chapters 3, 4, 11 and 13.

'I feel sad that at the start of my perimenopause journey I didn't have access to any information on the topic and I felt very alone, confused and misunderstood.'
Sarah Jones, Isle of Wight

CHAPTER 2

Benefits and Challenges

When menopause is making running hard, it can help to remember the benefits that running is going to give you. Let's begin with the positive news. You made a wonderful choice for your health when you decided to start running. Even if your running is minimal at the moment, it will still benefit you throughout menopause. Here are some of the ways that running and exercising regularly can help you in this life transition:

Reduces the risk of long-term health conditions: Our risk of contracting most diseases goes up as we get older and there's a sharp increase for many conditions around menopause. There's overwhelming evidence that exercising regularly helps to reduce our risk of almost all major diseases, including heart disease, type 2 diabetes and many types of cancer. The risk of dementia, depression and stroke are also lowered. The size of the risk reduction is generally over 20 per cent, which is huge and much higher than many medications prescribed to prevent diseases.

Lowers the risk of osteoporosis: Exercise is a perfect way to counteract the loss of bone density that accelerates around menopause. One in two women over 50 will fracture a bone due to osteoporosis, so this is really important.

Increases muscle mass: We can lose up to 1 per cent of our muscle mass each year from the age of 50. Muscles are vital to help us run and keep us healthy. The anti-inflammatories muscles produce when we use them directly lower our risk of many diseases. Running helps to preserve and build muscle mass.

Helps control weight: Being obese or overweight increases our risk of many health conditions and some menopause symptoms. While diet is the thing that most influences weight, exercise and movement definitely have a role to play too.

Improves balance and coordination: Falls are a leading cause of injury, disability and death worldwide. They're more common and severe in people over 60, but what we do now determines how likely we are to fall in the future. Exercise that helps our balance and coordination will reduce our risk of falls and increase the chances of us living independently in old age.

Helps reduce menopausal symptoms: Many menopause symptoms can be reduced by exercising regularly. From improving your sleep to easing joint pains, from potentially reducing hot flushes to helping control fatigue, being a runner is a gift during menopause.

Supports mental health: The boost in mood, the calmness and the general reset that a run gives is a bonus on any day, but when we're navigating change and challenge it's essential. Mental health symptoms are very common in menopause, so we're lucky to have the power of running to help us cope.

Improves social health: Having good social health improves our mental and physical health. Women often withdraw, and become more isolated and antisocial during menopause. Running connects us with others, whether it's running with a friend or belonging to a running community such as parkrun, it gives us the opportunity to interact with others and avoid becoming isolated or lonely which both have a negative impact on our health.

> 'I lost my dad to heart failure when he was 53. Post-menopausal women have a higher risk of heart conditions due to the drop in protective oestrogen, so at 50 I have decided that running is now a non-negotiable for me. I'm determined to stay active to maintain a strong cardiovascular system.'
>
> **Elaine Paterson,** London

WHY RUNNING IS SO GOOD IN MENOPAUSE

Running is the perfect exercise to do during menopause, not only for the hard medical benefits described above, but because running can be whatever you need it to be. You can work it around the unpredictability of how you're feeling. You can do a short, super-easy run when everything hurts, a sprint session when you feel full of power or a long, steady run to clear your mind. You can run with friends or alone, indoors or outdoors. It's hard to find another form of exercise that has such flexibility and this is key in menopause.

Running is also great, because it's easy to set goals. Even if the journey is up and down, working towards something can help you to stay positive and feel you are moving forwards at a time when everything might feel it's going backwards and spiralling downwards.

THE CHALLENGES

The impact that menopause has on your running might be mild or severe, short-lived or seemingly never-ending, but there are very few runners going through the hormonal changes of menopause who don't experience a negative effect on their running. Here are some of the challenges women face:

- Losing the love of running.
- Less motivation or drive to run.
- Losing running confidence.
- A decline in running performance.
- No progress in running.
- Menopause symptoms making running difficult.
- Not feeling the same benefits from running.

This sounds bleak, but it's the reality for the vast majority of women that I talk to. Changes to your running from menopause can start very insidiously, so you don't even really notice the difference, or very suddenly, when they literally stop you in your tracks. It can take a while before you link the changes in your running to your hormones. If your periods are haywire, it's an obvious symptom, but a subtle reduction in performance or a drop in running confidence isn't always such a clear connection.

> 'I started with perimenopausal symptoms at age 46. It really slowed down my running. It was harder for me to hit goal paces. I felt weighed down by the pounds that suddenly seemed to cling to me. I was so frustrated, yet I kept going back out to run. It was already so habitual by then that I wasn't going to let anything stop me doing what I love.'
> **Carri Ables**

What is it about the symptoms of menopause that cause them to have such an impact on running? I believe it's the following characteristics:

- Unpredictability – not knowing how you will feel day to day, or hour to hour.
- Severity – they can hit very hard.
- Nature – it's often new symptoms that you aren't used to dealing with.
- Extent – every system in the body can be affected.
- Uncontrollability – not being able to fully control the outcome.

If we're runners, then running is a constant in our lives; something we can turn to for help to manage the everyday strains of life. It's a time to relax, think and process events. It's also a way to challenge ourselves and gain personal growth. It gives us a sense of control. Throw in the characteristics of menopause symptoms and it's easy to see why the status quo is upset. Menopause disrupts the one thing in life that helps us to cope and brings us pleasure. Our running, our body and ultimately our life can feel out of control. It's easy to underestimate the impact this can have.

The impact of menopause symptoms

Menopause symptoms affect everyday life, but they can specifically impact running. We'll be looking at symptoms in detail in the following chapters. They can all be barriers to running and to keep going we need to find ways to reduce or remove them. For example, anxiety may make us not want to run on our own and feeling antisocial can put us off running with others. Breast pain can stop us sprinting and a dry, irritated vulva makes endurance running uncomfortable. Think about your own running and the impact your symptoms are having. Being aware of this impact is the first step in having some self-compassion and appreciating why running is hard for you right now.

The experience of menopause symptoms

You can't really predict how menopause will affect you and there are so many factors that influence your experience of it. There are, however, some known associations. For example, research has found that women with high levels of stress are more likely to experience worse hot flushes than those with lower stress levels.

> 'I've found that irregular periods, cramps, fatigue and niggles or injuries have had a huge negative effect on my running. However, it's also shown me how important it is to listen to my body and not worry about what others are doing. I might be slower and need to think more about recovery, but I can still run and take part in events. It's a great time to re-evaluate what running means for you.'
> **Sharon Flanagan,** Bolton

I mentioned earlier that women of different ethnicities can experience different menopause timing and they can experience symptoms in different ways, too. The British Menopause Society has created a tool for health professionals summarising the research and findings of the differences in menopause in ethnic minority women. This highlights that alongside an earlier average age of menopause, women of African-Caribbean descent experience a longer duration of symptoms. Hot flushes and night sweats are more frequent and severe, and sleep disruption is more common. They have more problems with weight gain and mental health issues, but are less likely to struggle with low libido. Women from Asia, for example from Japan and China, are less troubled by hot flushes, but more likely to have a low libido. They also get more muscle and joint pains, and suffer more with forgetfulness. Women from India and other parts of Asia have a much earlier average age of menopause and more vulval and bladder symptoms.

It's clear the challenges are big, but there's no doubt that the benefits are huge. This is such a crucial point in our lives to be active and running, so let's explore all these challenges and benefits, and make sure that we can gain from all that running has to offer us.

CHAPTER 3

Flushes and Sweats

Hot flushes, hot flashes, hot sweats – whatever you call them, they aren't pleasant. Around eight in 10 women get hot flushes or night sweats at some point during menopause. Every woman's experience is different, but they're commonly described as a warm sensation felt most intensely in the upper chest, neck and head, making you feel boiling hot, flushed and sweaty. When I was working as a GP, menopausal staff members would attempt to cool down by nipping into my room between patients to stand with their face directly under my air-conditioning unit.

With a night sweat, you wake up feeling really hot, often lying in a pool of sweat with soaking wet pyjamas and sheets. Then you become freezing cold and begin to shiver as your body tries to warm itself up again. Night sweats are exhausting for women who are badly affected.

Hot flushes and night sweats are known as vasomotor symptoms. *Vaso* comes from the Latin word *vās*, which means vessel, and *motor* which means movement. The vasomotor centre is responsible for narrowing or dilating your blood vessels to allow more or less blood to a particular part of your body. This is an important part of body temperature control, but more of that in a moment.

Although hot flushes are often the main symptom that comes to mind when menopause is mentioned, they aren't always the first thing that women notice. Only around half of women get hot flushes at the start of their perimenopause. They become more common and frequent as you progress through the transition, and they tend to peak close to the time of menopause itself. They do gradually decline in post-menopause, but while most women experience them for a total of four or five years, around 10 per cent of women are still having them 10 years or more post-menopause, albeit usually with less frequency and severity.

> 'In my twenties I had multiple surgeries and a chemical menopause to treat stage 4 endometriosis. I thought from these experiences I was somewhat prepared to deal with hot flashes later in life. I didn't expect to become a walking boiler I couldn't unplug. The heat and sweat were constant. Training for my tenth marathon was a disaster but somehow I found a way to get my heating system across the finish line.'
> **Julie W**

WHY DO YOU GET HOT FLUSHES AND NIGHT SWEATS?

The hypothalamus in the brain controls your body temperature. It's your internal thermostat. The body likes 'homeostasis' where everything is at a constant level. An even body temperature allows your body processes to perform optimally. When the hypothalamus senses your core body temperature rising, it starts a cascade of mechanisms to cool you down. These include:

- Making you sweat – when sweat evaporates off the skin, it takes heat with it.
- Flushing your skin – superficial blood vessels dilate to allow more blood to flow through them as blood loses heat to the outside when it travels close to the skin.
- Increasing your heart rate – this takes blood to the skin surface more quickly and rapidly circulates cooled blood.
- Increasing your breathing rate – heat is expelled in your breath and your oxygen intake increases as your body works harder to reduce its temperature.

It's a clever and effective thermoregulatory system, but during perimenopause the hypothalamus seems to get more sensitive to changes in body temperature. It accepts a narrower heat window and over-reacts or even fires up its cooling mechanisms inappropriately. There might also be more sensitivity and over-activity of peripheral blood vessels. The reasons behind all of this are not fully understood. Fluctuating oestrogen levels almost certainly play a role as there are oestrogen receptors in the brain and changes in oestrogen levels affect brain function. It's thought that FSH, which rises during perimenopause and remains high in post-menopause, could influence hot flushes, too, as well as varying levels of LH. There are a range of other brain chemicals and neurotransmitters that might also be involved. There is so much we don't understand, which is one of the reasons we don't have treatments that will guarantee to stop hot flushes – although HRT does a pretty good job in most women.

> 'I think being a runner meant I wasn't a stranger to feeling hot and sweaty so hot flushes were not as distressing.'
> **Colette,** Lancaster

GOOD TO KNOW

While there aren't any specific studies looking at the prevalence of hot flushes in runners compared to non-runners, it's interesting to look at the risk factors that are known to be associated with a higher incidence of hot flushes. These include obesity, a sedentary lifestyle and smoking, all of which are lower in runners than the general population. Therefore, it's fair to say that being a runner might put you at lower risk of being severely affected by hot flushes.

WHAT'S THE EFFECT ON RUNNING?

Here are some of the ways hot flushes and night sweats affect running:

- **Dehydration:** You can lose a significant amount of sweat through hot flushes and night sweats, and end up dehydrated, which has a knock-on effect on your running performance.

- **Poor sleep:** Being deprived of sleep due to frequent night sweats makes recovery harder and energy levels lower.
- **Temperature control:** Running feels harder if you're over-heating due to the extra effort your body is putting into lowering your temperature. It's also difficult to get your kit choice right.
- **Low motivation:** Choosing to get hot and sweaty in addition to menopause flushes isn't appealing. Motivation is also low if you're sleep deprived from night sweats.
- **Skin changes:** With extra sweating, skin is more prone to rashes and chafing. With the need to lose extra heat, your face might be redder during running and the redness lasts longer too.

> 'Everyone at running club laughs at me, because I always turn up in a vest, even on freezing cold days. I just get so unbearably hot when I run now.'
> **Cindy Phelps**

CAN RUNNING IMPROVE HOT FLUSHES?

Women who are regularly active tend to suffer less from menopausal symptoms than inactive women. While some studies have shown no improvement, or in some cases a worsening of hot flushes with exercise, particularly sudden bursts of high-intensity exercise, there's growing evidence that exercise itself can reduce the frequency and intensity of hot flushes, particularly if you're improving your fitness. When you become fitter, you improve your body's ability to regulate its temperature, and boost brain and skin circulation, which make your body more efficient at losing heat. It's always worth warming up thoroughly to gradually increase your body temperature. A regular habit of sustained, longer duration exercise is thought to be most beneficial in terms of managing hot flushes, so running is perfect.

HOW TO MANAGE HOT FLUSHES AND RUNNING

Here are six self-help tips for coping with hot flushes and minimising the impact they have on your running:

1. **Keep hydrated**: Get into the habit of drinking a glass of water when you wake up in the morning to counteract fluid lost during night sweats. Drink frequently on and off through the day, and especially before and after training.
2. **Avoid triggers**: Look for patterns to identify which lifestyle changes might reduce hot flushes. Alcohol, caffeine and spicy foods can trigger them, so can high-fat or high-sugar foods, in some women. Stress can be a flush trigger, but it's harder to avoid than a foodstuff.
3. **Go for layers**: Become the master of layering your running kit. You might need to put layers on and off several times during a run. Be flexible and go with what feels right for you, ignoring what everyone else is wearing.
4. **Keep cool**: Take steps to keep your core cool when you run. Choose cooler days, times and shadier routes; it's often colder at altitude. Windy days can make running harder, but might become your favourite as the wind cools you down. An iced drink before you run (this is called pre-cooling) can help and consider a small water spray to spritz your face. A hat will keep the sun off your head, but if you prefer to have that exposed to help lose heat, try a visor.
5. **Protect your skin**: Heavier sweating takes its toll on your skin. Wet clothes rub more than dry ones and chafing becomes common. Use skin lubricants such as Vaseline before you run and always shower soon after you finish. For more about skin changes during menopause see chapter 13.
6. **Sleep cool**: If your nights are interrupted by sweats, you need to take action. Avoid a hot drink right before bed. For more sleep tips see chapter 4.

WHEN THE SELF-HELP DOESN'T WORK

Vasomotor symptoms can be unbearable and have a huge impact on your life. I've seen women at their wits' end with sleep deprivation, considering leaving their jobs due to intense hot flushes. Please see your doctor if this is you – don't suffer in silence – because alongside the self-help measures, there are lots of other solutions:

Hormone replacement therapy (HRT): An extremely effective way to reduce hot flushes, for some women HRT is life-changing, for others it just makes things a bit more bearable. HRT is the first-line treatment for vasomotor symptoms, so if it's suitable for you to use and you want to do so, then it's the best and most effective first choice. For more about HRT, see chapter 15.

Non-hormonal treatments: There are alternatives to HRT that can reduce flushes, such as SSRIs, clonidine, gabapentin and pregabalin. These weren't specifically designed to be used to reduce flushes, but experience has shown this is one of their side-effects. SSRIs are antidepressants, clonidine is used for high blood pressure, and gabapentin and pregabalin are used as nerve painkillers and to treat epilepsy. This means they have other positive side-effects that might be helpful according to what your needs are, but similarly they can have effects, which some women don't want or can't tolerate. There's also a new drug called fezolinetant. This works directly on the temperature regulation centre in the brain. It's for the treatment of moderate or severe vasomotor symptoms in women who aren't able to use HRT, although at the time of writing it's only available as a private prescription. All of these options should be discussed with your doctor.

Cognitive behavioural therapy (CBT): CBT has been proven to be beneficial in reducing hot flushes in some women. This doesn't mean that hot flushes are all in our head or that we can always control them, but it does show that how we think has a direct effect on how our body reacts. CBT can also help to reduce anxiety and depression, which may be a cause or a result of hot flushes. It can improve stress levels and well-being, so whether that directly reduces hot flushes or helps you to manage them when they do happen, in my opinion that can only be a positive thing.

Supplements, herbal remedies and complementary therapies

There are many products that claim to help reduce hot flushes and night sweats. These include:

- Black cohosh
- Red clover
- Sage
- Vitamin E
- Soy
- Dong Quai (angelica)
- Agnus castus
- Evening primrose oil
- Angelic
- Ginseng
- St John's wort.

However, before you try any of these, please read chapter 15 which talks about the poor evidence and lack of regulation in the food supplement world. There are important things you need to consider before you start taking any of them, including how to do so safely.

> 'I sweat so much more when I run. I once had to take my contact lenses out mid-run, because the sweat was pouring down my forehead and into my eyes making them sting really badly.'
> **Tara,** Lancashire

When should I go to the doctor?

Hot flushes: There's a huge variation in the number of hot flushes women experience, ranging from one or two per week to 30 times a day. There is no 'normal' number or intensity that you have to put up with. Don't compare yourself to others. If they are impacting your day-to-day life or ability to do your job, to enjoy your hobbies (including running) or lowering your self-esteem, then take some action. Try the self-help tips above and see your doctor if these aren't helping.

Night sweats: Due to the sleep deprivation they cause, night sweats can have a big impact on your quality of life. If they're regularly interrupting your sleep and that's having a knock-on effect on your ability to live your life, then speak to your doctor. Although night sweats are common during menopause, they can sometimes happen for other reasons, including stress, as a side-effect of medication or due to medical conditions such as infection, diabetes or certain types of cancer. For this reason, if you have other symptoms along with regular night sweats, such as unexplained weight loss, a cough or swollen glands, then don't assume this is down to menopause. Make an appointment with your doctor.

Palpitations: Many women say they feel their heart racing, beating strongly or fluttering during a hot flush. Heart rate is controlled by the autonomic nervous system, which also deals with temperature regulation and is affected by fluctuating oestrogen levels. These sensations are called palpitations and around one in five menopausal women will experience them, often separately from flushes, although like flushes they can sometimes bring a feeling of anxiety or of mild breathlessness. They're more common if you have high stress levels and can be triggered by caffeine, alcohol and high sugar intake, so lifestyle changes can help minimise them. For me personally, ditching caffeine dramatically reduced my palpitations. HRT can be very effective for some women if oestrogen fluctuations are the main cause.

Although palpitations are usually harmless, they can feel scary and, because menopause isn't always the cause, you should see your doctor if:

- You have chest pain or tightness from your palpitations (call an emergency ambulance).

- You feel very short of breath, faint, dizzy or nauseated from your palpitations.
- You get palpitations when you exercise.
- You have palpitations most days.
- Your palpitations last more than a few minutes.
- Your heartbeat is jumping around in an irregular rhythm, whether that is fast, slow or normal speed.

'After my total hysterectomy, palpitations were waking me up at night. I couldn't work out if they were anxiety related or just another symptom of menopause. It never occurred to me that running could help but it did!'
Lisa Ruggles, Oxford

CHAPTER 4

Sleep

*M**enopause and the Workplace*, a report published by the Fawcett Society in 2022, revealed that 84 per cent of the 4014 menopausal British women surveyed found sleeping either somewhat or very difficult. A meta-analysis from 2023 revealed that just over 50 per cent of women around the world were affected by sleep disorders during menopause, with the highest levels being in post-menopause. It's always a spectrum, of course, from women who have minor, short-term sleep disturbances right through to those who have severe insomnia.

WHY DOES SLEEP MATTER?

Sleep is crucial for optimum body functioning. A lack of sleep can have long-term negative effects on your health and well-being, and lower your quality of life. It can increase your risk of chronic disease, lower your mood and reduce your ability to function. It can also mean you're more likely to struggle with your sex life.

Feeling exhausted can make running very difficult as sleep is vital for energy, recovery and running performance. Most runners don't sleep well the night before a big event, but what's more important are your longer-term sleep habits. When you sleep is when your body repairs, regenerates and reinforces itself; it's when you get fitter. Having a chronic sleep debt will wear you down physically and mentally, which won't help your running. You'll be more at risk of illness and injury, and won't recover or perform well.

WHY DO WOMEN SLEEP POORLY DURING MENOPAUSE?

Sleeping badly can encompass a range of sleep problems:

- Difficulty falling asleep.
- Waking up in the night.
- Waking early and not being able to go back to sleep.
- Poor quality sleep.

We don't fully understand all the reasons why menopause affects sleep, but we do know that waking frequently during the night is the most common menopausal sleep complaint. We need to remember, though, that sleeping patterns often change with age anyway. Older people tend to sleep less – melatonin is one of our sleep hormones and this reduces with age.

Sleep can be directly affected by menopause symptoms such as night sweats, but it can also be a problem in women who don't have nocturnal symptoms. This is most likely due to the complex interaction of sex hormone levels and brain chemicals. Studies have shown that decreasing oestrogen is associated with a higher chance of difficulty falling asleep in the first place and with staying asleep once you have dropped off. Progesterone makes some women drowsy, so it probably has a role in sleep pathways, too. Oestrogen and progesterone influence melatonin secretion in the brain. Melatonin is a hormone that your brain releases in the dark and it helps to regulate sleeping and waking. As oestrogen and progesterone levels reduce, melatonin secretion can fall. FSH may also be involved, as increasing FSH levels have been associated with greater odds of waking up several times during the night.

There have been a variety of studies looking at whether and how our sleep cycles, stages of sleep and brain wave activity alter as we move through menopause. While some have shown changes, there are so many variables that affect sleep other than changing hormone levels, it's hard to draw any concrete conclusions.

> 'Equipping myself with all the knowledge I can about menopause sleep symptoms has led to me to have a calming acceptance that this is just what happens. The less I stress about it, the quicker I fall back to sleep.'
>
> **Sarah Jones,** Isle of Wight

WHAT KEEPS WOMEN AWAKE?

Women who report a lot of hot flushes are more likely to have sleep disturbance, and those who have severe flushes are three times more likely to wake up frequently in the night, but the figure below shows the range of factors that can also affect sleep quality. It's easy to see why solving sleep problems isn't easy.

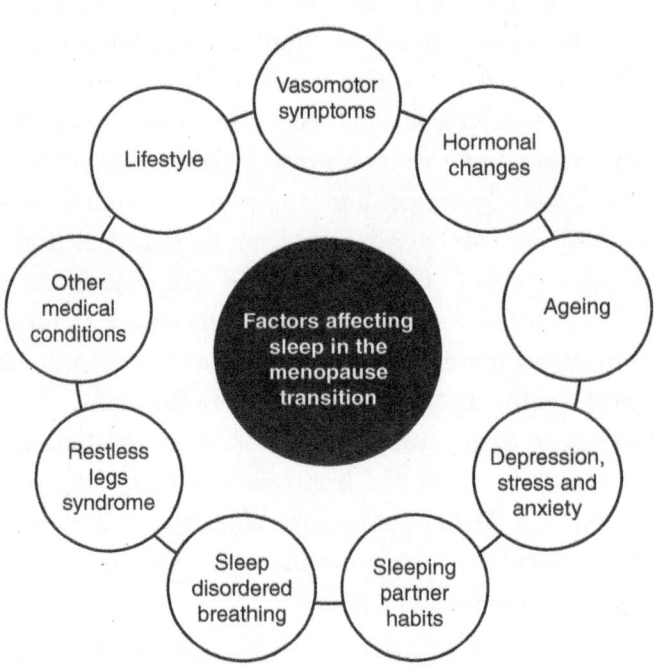

You need to get to the root cause of wakefulness, but it's often a variety of issues, many of which interact with each other. For example, poor sleep is often a result of stress and anxiety, which can trigger vasomotor symptoms. There are also a range of medical conditions that can affect sleep during menopause, including an overactive bladder and musculoskeletal problems, such as a frozen shoulder or hip pain.

Our sleep can be severely affected by the sleep habits and disorders of those we sleep next to as well. Sleep disordered breathing (SDB) includes snoring and upper-airway obstruction, and, while you may not have it yourself, your sleeping partner might and your sleep quality can be badly impacted. Interestingly, the risk of developing SDB becomes higher in post-menopause than pre-menopause. If you think you're having episodes of airway obstruction during the night, which presents with waking up gasping or snorting, it's important to see your doctor. SDB is underdiagnosed in women compared to men and it can result in a higher risk of cardiovascular disease.

Restless legs syndrome (RLS)

Restless legs mean an overwhelming need to move your legs. There can be associated cramps, involuntary jerks and a buzzing or tingling sensation in your legs. It usually happens at night, but it can be any time you're still, such as when sitting on an aeroplane. It can happen intermittently or regularly and severely disrupt sleep. It's not clear yet whether menopausal hormonal changes make RLS more likely and it may simply be related to getting older. The cause of it is unclear, but there can sometimes be an underlying medical condition, such as an underactive thyroid, iron deficiency or diabetes. Runners can experience restless legs after particularly hard or long runs.

Managing restless legs is tricky and severe cases may need medication. Treating underlying medical conditions will help to resolve it. Regular running might keep it away, but a run too close to bedtime or an intense or long run might set it off. Reducing caffeine and alcohol can help to prevent it and some women say taking magnesium or vitamin B6 helps them, although the research doesn't confirm that yet. If a bout strikes at night, try relaxation techniques and breathing through the urge to move your legs. If that isn't working, get up, stretch and massage your legs. If you're still fighting it, try a warm bath, heat pads or doing something completely different to distract you. It's horrible and if it's happening regularly, speak to your doctor.

> ### GOOD TO KNOW
>
> How much sleep you need varies from person to person, but sleep requirements tend to reduce with age. Most adults need around seven or eight hours to feel well and rested. Conversely, too much sleep is associated with higher rates of obesity. Regardless of how much sleep you normally get, factor in a little extra if you're training for an event, or generally working hard to improve your fitness, so you stay well and improve your recovery and performance.

HOW CAN I IMPROVE MY SLEEP?

To resolve sleep problems, begin by identifying the causes of your sleep disturbance. Which of the factors on page 30 are affecting you? It can be a big jumble to begin with, but consider how they interact and whether one is affecting another. Keeping a sleep diary can help you spot any patterns and triggers.

As with all menopausal symptoms, begin by controlling what you can control. Establish habits that help your body clock switch on and off at the correct time. The list of things you can try is long, dull and all take a bit of effort. You may have heard them before, but they can still make a difference. Pick one and once that's become routine for you, add a second, then a third and so on.

Healthy sleep habits

- **Avoid caffeine:** The Sleep Foundation recommends avoiding caffeine for at least eight hours before you go to bed. How long caffeine stays in your system varies according to your genetics, weight, and how much and how frequently you drink it. Even if you're someone who can fall asleep straight after a cup of coffee, it can still affect your sleep quality. Remember, caffeine is also in tea, chocolate and some fizzy drinks, as well as some sports energy gels and drinks.

- **Avoid alcohol**: Alcohol, even in small amounts, is well known to affect sleep quality. It might help you get off to sleep, but you're likely to wake up frequently in the night as your sleep becomes shallower. Alcohol can also be a trigger for night sweats. The Sleep Foundation recommends avoiding alcohol for at least three hours before you go to bed, so weigh up whether that glass of wine is worth it.
- **Look after your bladder**: Sometimes it's the need to pee that wakes you up (for more about bladder issues, see chapter 8). Most women don't drink enough fluids, but try to drink plenty throughout the day, so you're not drinking loads before bed. Also, minimise alcohol and caffeine, which can irritate your bladder.
- **Set your alarms**: Go to bed and get up at the same time every day, including the weekends. Avoid naps, but if you really need one, then make it no more than 30 minutes and not too late in the day.
- **Wind down**: Create your own pre-sleep ritual. That could be reading, gentle yoga or listening to music. Meditation, massage and journaling can all help you to relax. Do the same thing every night, so it becomes a set routine that lets your body know sleep is next.
- **Get outside**: Daylight on your face in the morning will help you sleep at night, so open the door and step outside, ideally within half an hour of waking. Take a quick walk or sit outside for your morning cuppa.
- **Go screen free**: The blue light from screens makes your brain think it's still daytime because the sun emits blue light. During the day it makes you feel alert, but before bed it affects your circadian rhythm and natural sleep-wake cycle. The jury is out as to the effectiveness of wearing blue-light-blocking glasses to improve sleep quality, but if you can don't look at a screen, including TV, for at least two hours before bedtime.

- **Create a sanctuary**: Keep your bedroom cool, dark and quiet. Use it as a sanctuary of sleep. If you work from home, try not to work in your bedroom.
- **Exercise**: People who exercise regularly sleep better than those that don't. Going out for a run during the day also gives you that important daylight exposure. However, running too close to bedtime can make it difficult to fall asleep, so you might need to change your run time or do some serious winding down afterwards.

> 'Night sweats and early-morning waking, both can get in the bin. My sleep is better with HRT, but it's still triggered by wine, even one glass, and sugary food in the evening.'
> **Anonymous**

When should I go to the doctor?

Sleep problems: The cause and severity of your sleep problems determines how long you should persevere with self-help and when you should go and see the doctor. For example, if your night sweats are frequently disturbing your sleep or you think your lack of sleep may come from being depressed, then don't wait around. Similarly, if you have very restless legs, sleep disordered breathing or think there may be a medical condition underlying your lack of sleep, start the lifestyle changes, but make an appointment with your doctor, too.

If despite trying your best to improve your sleep it has not improved and has been disturbed over a number of months, then make an appointment. Good sleep is very important for a good quality of life, so don't suffer in silence.

TREATMENTS FOR SLEEP PROBLEMS

Thankfully there are some effective treatments you can access via your doctor when the self-help hasn't helped.

CBT: A psychological treatment, CBT helps you think, feel and act differently in order to change the way you cope with a particular problem. When CBT is used for insomnia, it's called CBT-I. CBT-I can be very effective in treating sleep problems in menopause, regardless of whether you have vasomotor symptoms or not. If night sweats have been reduced by HRT, but sleep problems persist, try CBT-I. There may be waiting lists to access it, but there have been good results with online courses.

HRT: When it comes to hot flushes and night sweats HRT can be transformational, and it can help other symptoms that might be keeping you awake, such as bladder or vulval problems. Some women who use micronised progesterone as part of their HRT (see chapter 15) find it makes them feel drowsy, so they take it at night. Not every woman whose vasomotor symptoms are reduced by HRT sleeps well; they can still have wakeful nights. Identify any other factors that could be contributing to poor sleep and do your best to create healthy sleep habits.

> 'My sleep has been affected for a considerable number of years due to night sweats. I went on HRT because my work was affected by lack of sleep. This helped although I still suffer from sleep disturbance most nights.'
> **Jude,** Lancaster

Other medications

After a discussion, your doctor might recommend other medications to resolve your sleep problems. For example, gabapentin or low-dose antidepressants, used to reduce hot flushes when HRT isn't suitable, can also help sleep. Sleeping tablets are not recommended, because they should only ever be used in the short term, you can become dependent on them very quickly and they aren't suitable for the longer-term sleep problems associated with menopause. Similarly, there's not enough evidence yet to recommend melatonin as a long-term treatment. It can certainly help reset your body clock if you have jetlag, but it's not currently thought to be an effective option for insomnia in menopause.

Supplements

Alongside supplements to help reduce night sweats, some women take a range of supplements to try to help them sleep. These include magnesium, valerian, 5-HTP and L-Theanine. More scientific evidence is needed before these can be fully recommended as treatments (see chapter 15).

> 'I found sleeping was greatly interrupted, and I often got up and went for a short run, and then went back to bed. Doing this stopped me lying in bed getting frustrated and fed up!'
> **Maggie Lightfoot**

CHAPTER 5

Energy Levels

Feeling tired all the time and having no energy is common during menopause. Just getting through the day can be a challenge and running can feel impossible. Sometimes you're just not firing on all cylinders, at others you're completely knocked off your feet. It might be a daily grind or something that happens intermittently and it might affect you physically, mentally or both. Low energy levels are frustrating and challenging.

When it comes to running, figuring out what's tiredness and what's lack of motivation can be tricky. Knowing whether a run will make you feel better and energise you or will deplete your energy stores further isn't always obvious. Sometimes we don't run because we feel tired and then we beat ourselves up about not going. It's tough and we can be really hard on ourselves.

In this chapter we'll explore some of the reasons you might be knackered. It's unlikely to be just one thing, it's usually a combination of factors. You might not be able to control them all, but there may be some that you can influence. We'll begin with menopause symptoms and lifestyle factors that can affect our energy levels and move on to medical conditions that cause fatigue.

MENOPAUSE SYMPTOMS

Many menopause symptoms can make you tired. The obvious one is disrupted sleep (see chapter 4). You might find your tolerance for missing sleep diminishes and a late night can take days to get over. It's not just poor sleep though, because aches and pains, recurrent hot flushes or brain fog all drain your battery, and high anxiety levels and low mood are exhausting.

In addition to menopause symptoms causing fatigue, it's also thought that the falling levels of oestrogen, progesterone and testosterone directly affect our energy levels through their interaction with the brain and thyroid gland, which both control metabolism.

LIFESTYLE

Lifestyle is the number one cause of low energy levels. I don't mean partying or burning the candle at both ends, although if you're doing that, then of course you'll feel tired. I'm talking about the basics of what we do each day and the implication of what goes on in our wider world.

> 'I've really learned to listen to my own body, which I never did before. I understand when I need to rest and I feel empowered to say no, because I'm kind to myself first.'
> **Susan Reynolds,** Harrogate

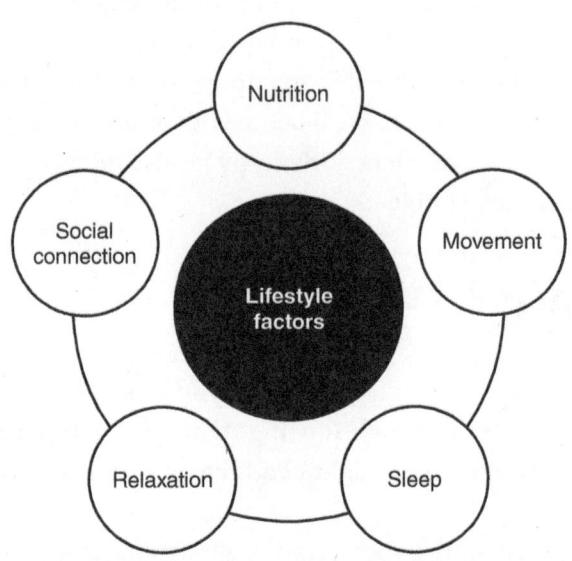

Nutrition

We get our energy from food. A calorie is a unit of energy and insufficient calorie intake results in low energy levels. The timing of your eating and the foods that make up your calorie intake are important in maintaining energy levels. Many women are low in energy because they simply don't eat enough or what and when they eat doesn't serve their needs. This is very true for runners, who expend more energy than non-runners and need readily available energy to fuel a run. You might jump on a caffeine or sugar rollercoaster in an attempt to increase your energy, but the highs and lows can make you feel awful and even more tired. For more about how to fuel your body for consistent energy, see chapter 16.

Movement

A run can recharge you, but it can also make you tired, especially if you're moving through an incremental training plan to improve your fitness. Exercise can feel harder to do and take longer to recover from during menopause. You might run less if other areas of your life are using all your energy. If you prioritise running, you'll have less energy to give to work or family. You might even end up overtraining in a bid to escape or to prove yourself. It helps to be open to your relationship with running changing for a while and to adapting what you do. For more about managing your training in menopause, see chapter 17.

> 'I seem full of energy when I'm moving around. I feel fine when I'm running, walking or biking, but as soon as I stop or sit down I immediately turn into granny mode. It feels like my whole system slows down, mind, body and spirit. Motion is lotion for sure.'
> **Elaine Paterson,** London

Sleep

As mentioned, sleep can be hard to come by in menopause and has a direct effect on energy levels, so we need to prioritise it and be disciplined with self-help measures. If you really can't sleep, it's good to know that just lying still and relaxing tops up your energy levels, and is still restorative for your body.

Relaxation

The pressures on women are high, but much of this comes from societal expectations. Around the average age of menopause, women are often at the peak of their careers in jobs with high levels of responsibility, and they may be caring for children and elderly parents, too. You might have big life changes such as becoming an empty nester or grieving the death of parents. If you have a premature menopause, the life events running alongside your menopause can be completely different or you might be grieving an early loss of your fertility. Aside from coping with menopause symptoms, there's so much else going on in the lives of women that takes energy.

Think about all the things you do in an average week and all the things on your mind. If each of those things was an item you packed into a rucksack, how big or heavy would yours be? Some women are walking happily with a small pack that gets a bit bigger from time to time, but they put things in and take things out, and can stride out without too much difficulty. Others have an enormous pack which is so heavy they can barely walk. They need to keep stopping and resting, and moving forwards takes so much energy. How big is your rucksack? Is it any wonder you're tired?

Giving ourselves time to relax is one of the most important things we can do if we're lacking in energy. It's easy to underestimate the effect that stress has on us. Doing something that allows you to forget about all the tabs open in your brain and put your rucksack down for a bit will reduce fatigue. Choose something that distracts you and completely absorbs you, even for a short time. You know what will suit you, but here are some things that work for me:

- A trail run where I have to focus on tricky terrain.
- A run in the woods or forest, which is so calming.
- Watching a film, ideally in a cinema so I can't do anything but watch it.
- Seeing a friend who makes me laugh.
- A challenging weights session where all my attention has to be on form and effort.
- A few deep breaths with my eyes closed.

In menopause, you might have reactions or see changes in your coping levels that are new to you. It's important to know that even a few minutes of relaxation here and there will help. Try an emergency brain break, such as a few deep breaths, when you feel stress building up.

> 'I experience a lot of fatigue in between my bursts of energy, although I can push myself if I need to. The backlash is days of tiredness.'
> **Hilary**

Social connection

Some people are refreshed by being with others, some are reinvigorated by time on their own. Social health is an important part of everyone's general health, but it doesn't have to mean spending lots of time with lots of people. Too much time with others or with the wrong people could be contributing to your low energy levels. Similarly, too much time on your own could be a trigger for your fatigue. It's getting the balance right for you that counts.

You might not have considered your social connections as a cause of your fatigue, but it's worth reflecting on who you spend your time with and whether those relationships are energy sapping or energy filling. What can you do to spend less time with the former and more time with the latter? Remember, too, that friends and family can help to share the load in your rucksack. Be proactive and ask them to help lighten your load. Likewise, be wary of people who keep giving you things from their rucksack and expecting you to carry them, especially if there's no sign of them taking them back. It's okay to say no, often.

MEDICAL CONDITIONS

It's wrong to assume that fatigue and lack of energy are always down to hormones and lifestyle. There are also important medical conditions that can cause excessive tiredness.

Anaemia

Red blood cells transport oxygen around the body. When red cell numbers are low, it's called anaemia and the symptoms are a result of the body trying its best to get oxygen from the lungs to tissues and organs. Anaemia generally happens quite slowly and while non-runners might not be aware of it until it gets quite severe, as a runner, particularly one that monitors stats, you're probably going to notice it sooner. You might notice:

- Your resting heart rate is higher.
- Your average heart rate is higher on your runs.
- Your VO2 max is decreasing.
- You're more out of breath when you run or when you walk upstairs.
- You feel light-headed, dizzy or get palpitations.
- You keep getting slower and more out of breath on your usual route.

When it comes to perimenopause, there are two main causes of anaemia to consider. Firstly, if you have heavier or more frequent periods in your perimenopause, then you might be losing blood more quickly than your body can make it, resulting in a lower number of red cells in your bloodstream. Secondly, if your body doesn't have the building blocks it needs to make the red cells, then production is low. Iron is needed to make red cells and iron deficiency is the most common cause of anaemia in the UK. You might not be getting enough iron in your diet or not be absorbing it from your gut properly if you have a condition such as coeliac disease or inflammatory bowel disease. If you've got heavy periods, your body might be using up all your iron stores as it constantly tries to replace the red cells that are being lost during bleeding. Runners have higher iron requirements than non-runners, and it's easy to quietly slip into iron deficiency if you're training hard and not making extra effort to eat enough iron. If not addressed, iron deficiency can lead to anaemia.

Iron deficiency anaemia is treated by raising iron levels by increasing dietary iron and, if necessary, taking an iron supplement, but it's important to look for and treat the cause. That might mean looking at ways to reduce the amount of period blood you're losing (see chapter 6). Crucially, if you do have iron deficiency, you should be seeing a doctor who may order tests and investigations to find the reason for it. For example, your low iron levels could be caused by a dietary issue or even a serious condition such as bowel cancer, where blood can be lost silently in your stool. Treatment with iron needs to be continued until anaemia is reversed and then continued for another couple of months to replenish iron stores (iron is stored in the body as ferritin). You may be advised to continue taking an iron supplement long term.

Folate and B12 are also needed for red cell production and a deficiency in these can also cause anaemia. This type of anaemia is rarer and usually due to problems absorbing these vitamins or hereditary conditions. Vegans and vegetarians are at higher risk of B12 deficiency, so it's a good idea to take a daily B12 supplement if you follow a meat-free diet (see chapter 16).

Thyroid disorders

Your thyroid gland is in the front of your neck and it plays an important role in metabolism. An under- or overactive thyroid can cause fatigue and both conditions become more common around menopause. As shown in the following table, there's a lot of crossover with menopause symptoms, so it can be very confusing.

Overactive thyroid (hyperthyroidism)	Underactive thyroid (hypothyroidism)
Fatigue	Fatigue
Irritability	Weight gain
Anxiousness or feeling on edge	Constipation
Heat intolerance and sweating	Dry skin and thinning hair
Palpitations	Low mood
Disturbed sleep	Slow thinking
Reduced number of periods	Irregular or heavy periods

Hypothyroidism affects around 1 to 2 per cent of people in the UK, 10 times more women than men and gets more frequent with age. Over the age of 60, 10 to 20 per cent of women have an underactive thyroid. Most cases of hypothyroidism are due to an autoimmune condition (Hashimoto's disease) where the immune system starts recognising the thyroid cells as harmful, attacking them and damaging the gland. Iodine is needed to make thyroid hormones and iodine deficiency is a common cause of hypothyroidism around the world, but it's rare in the UK. Your thyroid can also become underactive if you have previously been treated for hyperthyroidism or as a side-effect of certain medications. The exact links between hypothyroidism and menopause aren't really understood, but we know that women who have POI are more likely to have autoimmune thyroid disease, so there's clearly an interplay between the different hormonal systems.

Treatment involves taking daily thyroid replacement tablets containing thyroxine, the main hormone that is being underproduced by the gland. The dose you need is very individual and can change, so it requires monitoring by regular blood tests. Hypothyroidism is usually managed by your GP.

Hyperthyroidism affects around 0.5 to 1 per cent of people in the UK. Like hypothyroidism, it's 10 times more likely in women than men and again it's most commonly caused by an autoimmune condition (Grave's disease). Nodules can form on the gland or the gland can become inflamed, resulting in the overproduction of thyroid hormones. It's important to spot hyperthyroidism, because, if left untreated, it can cause eye disease, pregnancy problems or, rarely, a 'thyroid storm', where blood pressure suddenly shoots up to life-threatening levels. Treatment for hyperthyroidism is usually directed by a specialist (endocrinologist) and includes taking medication to suppress the gland, having radioiodine therapy to destroy thyroid tissue or having surgery to remove part or all of the gland.

> ### GOOD TO KNOW
>
> HRT will help symptoms that are caused by menopause. If your symptoms are caused by a thyroid disorder, this condition needs to be treated and stabilised in the appropriate way. A thyroid disorder may be making your menopausal symptoms worse and treating it may ease them. Interestingly, if you're already being treated for hypothyroidism, the amount of thyroxine you need can change when you hit perimenopause. It can also change if you start taking oestrogen HRT in tablet form, but it won't be affected by oestrogen HRT that's absorbed via the skin. If your thyroid symptoms are worsening or changing, speak to your doctor, who can arrange a blood test and tweak the dose of your thyroxine if necessary.

MENTAL HEALTH PROBLEMS

Mental health conditions affect our energy levels just as much as, if not more than, physical ones. There isn't an easy measure, such as a red blood cell level, to make the diagnosis, determine severity or monitor progress, but it doesn't make them any less important. Both anxiety and depression can cause extreme tiredness. This can be due to their effect on sleep, but sometimes sleep is excessive and the fatigue is severe. A certain level of stress in our lives is to be expected, but long term or severe stress can trigger anxiety and depression. If you think your lack of energy may be down to a mental health condition, it needs treating so you can regain your energy. For more about mental health in menopause, see chapter 14.

GOOD TO KNOW

Adrenal fatigue is not a condition recognised by conventional medicine. The theory is that after periods of extreme stress the adrenal glands burn out from overproducing large amounts of cortisol. This is then blamed for a group of symptoms, including tiredness, weight gain and salt or sugar cravings. The Endocrine Society is clear that there is no scientific evidence to support this theory and there is no test to diagnose it, as cortisol levels are normal in adrenal fatigue. The symptoms are generalised and common in many recognised medical conditions and shouldn't be attributed to adrenal fatigue.

Expensive and complicated vitamin regimes, and herbal and hormonal supplements, are offered for adrenal fatigue. There may be some initial improvement of symptoms due to a placebo effect and because giving anyone a bit of steroid will make them feel good, but there is no evidence of long-term benefit and some treatments may be dangerous. It's wise to question the credibility of anyone diagnosing you with adrenal fatigue and never self-diagnose.

Note that 'adrenal fatigue' is not the same as adrenal insufficiency, which is a recognised condition, diagnosed by blood tests which show low cortisol levels, and requiring ongoing cortisol replacement.

OTHER MEDICAL CONDITIONS

Both chronic fatigue syndrome (CFS), also called myalgic encephalomyelitis (ME), and long Covid can both present with extreme fatigue. This book is not the place for a detailed description of the diagnosis and management of them, but I wanted to mention them as some of the symptoms cross over with menopause. Headaches, muscle pains and dizziness are common, so are brain fog, disrupted sleep and poor temperature control. I've seen women on their knees before they ask for help. When fatigue is severe or prolonged, discuss it with a doctor to check whether other medical conditions could be the cause.

When to see your doctor

It's important to know that certain medical conditions which are more common in midlife can present with low energy and we need to be careful not to attribute everything to menopause. How on earth do you know what is what? If your energy levels are low, the first thing to do is to address your lifestyle, and improve and control all the things you can. See your doctor if:

- Lifestyle changes are not helping your symptoms.
- Your symptoms are severe, sudden or progressive in nature.
- You have a family history of under- or overactive thyroid conditions.
- You think you may be anaemic – do you have heavy periods, shortness of breath on exertion or a raised pulse rate?
- You are under 45 – it's important to identify whether you're having an early menopause.
- You have unexplained weight loss, palpitations or tremor.
- You started HRT for your symptoms, but there has been no improvement or they have got worse.

In these situations, alongside talking to you and examining you, your doctor will most likely request some blood tests to identify if there is something more than lifestyle-related fatigue and perimenopause going on.

MANAGING YOUR ENERGY LEVELS

Our energy levels are dependent on many factors and it's vital that we look at the bigger picture of our lives to see where our energy is going. Once we do this, we can identify what we can influence and change. Managing energy levels is an ongoing and daily task. Running can help to energise us, but it can sometimes add to our life load. If you're wanting to run more, get fitter or aim for a race, it's essential to look at what is going on in life, and plan your expectations and training accordingly.

Something has to give to allow you more energy for running. What can you share, delegate or do without? Listening to your body becomes important. Sometimes it's okay to run when you're a bit tired as long as you aren't putting pressure on yourself to pull out a PB. On another day you might be better to give it a miss. Only you can answer that question, but you may have to get it wrong a few times to find out. Learn from your mistakes. Be honest with yourself about whether you are making an excuse, lacking motivation or deep down you know you should rest, and do that, guilt free.

> 'I've found that I have to really listen to my body, rather than trying to stick to generic training plans, as fatigue has made running quite hard. Accepting that hiking is still good training for longer distances has really helped me adapt my training.'
>
> **Emma Davies,** South Wales

CHAPTER 6

Periods

Lots of women look forward to menopause, because they will be free from periods. Women have an average of 450 periods in their lifetime and that's a lot, especially if your periods are problematic. Let's face it, even if they aren't heavy or painful, periods can still be a nuisance, especially for runners. As I mentioned in the introduction, menopause is not always a joyous time, because the end of periods marks the end of fertility and this can be a difficult thing to come to terms with. It's also important to bear in mind that your periods stopping is not always due to perimenopause and active women in particular need to be aware of other reasons this might happen.

A change in your periods may be the first sign that you're entering perimenopause, but that's not always the case. Sometimes other symptoms, particularly mental health symptoms, such as anxiety, come first. Before periods stop completely, they usually go haywire. In the perimenopause you might experience a change in:

- Cycle length, with more frequent or less frequent periods.
- Bleeding amount, with heavier or lighter periods.
- Length of bleed, with longer or shorter periods.
- Period pain, with more cramping and discomfort.

CAUSES OF HEAVY AND PAINFUL PERIODS IN PERIMENOPAUSE

It's important to consider the causes of heavy, painful or irregular bleeding, before just cracking on with managing it. There are conditions that affect periods at any time in your reproductive life, but may persist, flare up or even begin in perimenopause.

- **Dysfunctional uterine bleeding (DUB):** This is the commonest reason for heavy periods and is the term used when there is no other cause. It may be a result of the fluctuating hormone levels of perimenopause. Some cycles become anovulatory cycles, when no egg is released, and just like when periods began at menarche, these are typically irregular and heavy.
- **Endometriosis:** In endometriosis, endometrial tissue which lines the uterus is found in other places, such as on the ovaries, fallopian tubes, bladder or bowel. The tissue behaves like the uterus lining so causes pain and bleeding. During perimenopause, women with endometriosis often find the hormonal fluctuations make their symptoms flare up. Eventually, when periods end, these symptoms reduce or stop, but 2 to 5 per cent of women with endometriosis still experience symptoms in post-menopause.
- **Adenomysosis:** Endometrial tissue grows within the muscle layers of the uterus (myometrium) and when it bleeds, the blood gets trapped between the layers causing cramps and pelvic pain. Like endometriosis, perimenopause can exacerbate this condition.
- **Polycystic ovary syndrome:** PCOS is a complex condition affecting two in 10 women. It can cause irregular periods, mood swings and changes to hair and skin, so it can be difficult to differentiate from perimenopause. The additional fluctuations of hormones during perimenopause can make PCOS symptoms worse.
- **Uterine polyps:** These are small overgrowths of endometrial tissue. You're most likely to develop them in your forties or fifties, which is around the perimenopause for most women. They can cause irregular or heavy periods and bleeding between periods, too. They're usually benign (non-cancerous), but can be removed if it is felt there is a high risk of them becoming cancerous.
- **Fibroids:** Fibroids are benign tumours that grow in the uterus and the most common type grows into the muscle wall. Fibroids are made of a mixture of muscle cells and fibrous tissue. They are extremely common and it's estimated that 70 to 80 per cent of women will have a fibroid at some point during their lives.

Women of African-Caribbean descent are three times more likely to have fibroids than white women and their fibroids grow more quickly, tend to be bigger and cause more severe symptoms. Asian women have an increased risk, too. Fibroids tend to arise before perimenopause starts, but they can appear during it. They frequently cause heavy, long and painful periods. Bloating, constipation and painful sex are common, too. They usually shrink after menopause, but may continue to grow, especially in black women of African descent. Fibroids may need to be monitored if you start HRT, because the oestrogen element of it can cause them to enlarge.

- **Endometrial hyperplasia:** This is thickening of the lining of the uterus, which can lead to heavy or irregular periods and bleeding between periods. It happens when oestrogen levels are not balanced by progesterone levels, so is more common if you are overweight, have PCOS or are using HRT without a sufficient dose of progestogen. It's also more common in women who have diabetes or are taking tamoxifen for breast cancer. Some types of endometrial hyperplasia are unlikely to turn into cancer, but others, called atypical hyperplasia, have a higher risk, so a biopsy (sample) of the tissue is taken to be examined under the microscope.
- **Infection:** Infections of the pelvis, including sexually transmitted infections, such as chlamydia, can cause pelvic inflammatory disease and heavy periods.
- **Other medical conditions or medications:** Disorders that affect blood clotting, or medications such as warfarin that thin the blood, can result in heavy bleeding. An underactive thyroid gland can also cause heavy periods.

'I've had three surgeries for longstanding stage three endometriosis and it has a habit of coming back aggressively. At first I thought running made it worse, then I realised it's a certain style of running. If I'm sticking to a strict training plan, putting pressure on myself and running hard, fast or long kilometres, it stresses my body.

If I go for a fun-focused trail run and walk combination, and just relax and enjoy myself, it doesn't send me into a pain flare. It's taken a bit to get to the point of figuring this out using trial and error, and listening to my body.'

Hazel, New Zealand

> ## GOOD TO KNOW
>
> Having a normal menstrual cycle is a marker of good health. Cycles naturally become disrupted in perimenopause and stop in post-menopause, so we lose this guide. This is a really important time to be developing other ways to monitor our health such as our energy levels, sleep and blood pressure.

MANAGING HEAVY PERIODS

Menorrhagia is the medical term for heavy periods. There are various definitions as to how much blood loss counts as heavy, but all that really matters is whether your bleeding is too heavy for you. If it's stopping you being able to live your normal life, because you have to keep changing tampons and pads or you're flooding through clothes, then it's too heavy, regardless of the actual millilitres of blood lost. There are too many women coping with excessive bleeding, because they've been led to think that's just part of being a woman, but please speak to your doctor, because there are plenty of things that can be done.

Most of us get used to managing our running around our periods and have done so for years, so it's very frustrating if things suddenly change in perimenopause. You can find you're running less, racing less and generally being less active as a result of your perimenopausal periods. The impact of this on your physical and mental health shouldn't be underestimated.

Practical options

We get stuck in our ways with period products, but be open-minded. Consider trying something different such as a menstrual cup, which can hold more blood than a tampon. Period underwear is a wonderful invention, either on its own or as a back-up to a tampon. There are some nice styles, which vary in how much blood they hold, so you can choose what suits you best. When it comes to running kit, boring black is best if you're worried about leaking blood, but you could invest in a skort or a running dress to hide bulky pads. It's also worth getting a decent running belt, vest or pack to hold period products.

Non-hormonal options

Taking non-steroidal anti-inflammatories (NSAIDs), such as ibuprofen, regularly through a period can reduce blood flow by up to a third in some women. Check with your pharmacist to make sure you don't have any contraindication to taking them. Mefenamic acid is another option, but in the UK this is only available on prescription from your doctor. It's important to know that NSAIDs aren't recommended within 48 hours of doing an endurance event, such as a marathon, due to the increased risk of kidney damage when you are dehydrated. Tranexamic acid is a medication taken during your period to reduce the amount of blood lost. It can be very effective, but isn't suitable for everyone and needs to be prescribed by your doctor.

Hormonal options

An intrauterine system (IUS) is a coil, which slowly releases synthetic progestogen into the womb and, for the vast majority of women, results in light or no periods after three to six months. This is the most effective way to manage heavy bleeding in perimenopause. A small number of women develop irregular or heavy bleeding and it doesn't suit them, but when it works, it can be a game-changer. It's also a great contraceptive and it can be used as the progestogen element of HRT, so it's a good choice for this time of life. Again, be open-minded. Just because it didn't suit your friend doesn't mean it won't suit you.

Combined oral contraceptive pills (COCPs) are an effective way to manage heavy periods in pre-menopause and can be helpful in perimenopause, too. They suppress ovulation and smooth out hormonal fluctuations. They're usually only prescribed up to age 50, due to increased risks of blood clots and cardiovascular disease over this age.

Progestogen contraceptives, such as the progestogen-only pill (POP), Depo-Provera injection or progestogen implant can help to manage heavy bleeding, although the latter two only tend to be used if contraception is needed as well. There are pros and cons to each, so you need a careful discussion with your doctor. Progestogen tablets called norethisterone, used in the second half of the menstrual cycle, are sometimes used to reduce bleeding, but they aren't as effective as other options, don't work as contraception and aren't suitable for everyone. They're usually a short-term, rescue measure. Medroxyprogesterone is an alternative sometimes used by doctors.

You can still use HRT if you're having periods; it's a myth that you have to wait until they've stopped. If you're starting HRT to manage other menopause symptoms, it can help to regulate your periods. If you're already on HRT and your periods become heavy, speak to your doctor about making changes to your dose or the way you take your HRT. For a detailed look at HRT, see chapter 15.

> 'I developed extremely heavy periods which led to low iron levels. I had no energy and couldn't run for several months. I had a Mirena coil fitted and this has been a real game-changer for me.'
> **Kerry**

Other options

If the practical, non-hormonal and hormonal options don't work, there are still more heavy-duty measures to try, but you need to be referred to a gynaecologist to discuss and access these. They include using medications that switch off the ovaries and put the body into a menopausal state, often called a 'chemical menopause'. An endometrial ablation, where the lining of the womb is removed, is another option. Finally, you may be offered a hysterectomy, which is an operation to remove the uterus completely.

> ## GOOD TO KNOW
>
> Norethisterone can be used to delay or postpone a period, for example if your period is due on race day. However, it's not suitable for everyone due to an increased risk of blood clots in the legs and lungs, and in terms of running it's not guaranteed to stop your bleeding. Also, be aware it may make you feel bloated or sluggish and affect your performance.

CONSEQUENCES OF HEAVY PERIODS

Managing heavy periods isn't just about stopping blood from leaking, it's about the wider impact of blood loss, which can affect your physical and mental health. Heavy periods can cause anaemia (see chapter 5). Your life can become more restricted if you have heavy or irregular bleeding. You can find yourself becoming nervous about being far from home, feel vulnerable at work or struggle to run. This is at a time when you may be experiencing mood changes, anxiety and a lack of self-confidence from the hormonal swings of perimenopause. Combine all this and it's easy to understand the negative effects of heavy perimenopausal bleeding.

Keeping track of when you bleed and how you feel can help you manage your periods. There may not be a pattern if your cycle becomes irregular, but you can still get an overview of what's going on. You might see the bleeding time getting shorter or the gaps between periods getting longer. You will also be able to identify when you haven't had a period for 12 consecutive months and have reached menopause. It becomes easier to spot if there is abnormal bleeding and it gives you a clearer picture to explain to your doctor.

Painful periods

The impact of painful periods can be wildly underestimated. Pain can be debilitating, even when blood flow is light. It can begin before bleeding starts and continue until bleeding stops. Painful periods (dysmenorrhoea) are caused by cramping of the muscular wall of the uterus. The muscles contract to help shed the endometrium, but this contraction squashes the small blood vessels, which supply the muscles, and further cramping results. A degree of discomfort is to be expected, but being in pain every month is not a normal part of being a woman. Too many women are suffering. There may be an underlying cause such as endometriosis, adenomyosis or fibroids, but often there isn't.

Reducing the number and frequency of periods is one way to reduce the pain, so check the hormonal methods for heavy periods already discussed. In terms of relieving pain, heat and exercise can both help, but painkillers are probably your best bet. NSAIDs, such as ibuprofen, are the most effective at reducing period pain, but not everyone can take them, so check with your pharmacist and remember they aren't the best choice for long endurance runs. Paracetamol is safer, but may not be as good at easing the pain. Speak to your doctor if over-the-counter painkillers are not helping.

A LACK OF PERIODS

It's not just heavy and painful periods that are important – a lack of periods (amenorrhoea) matters, too. Not having a period might feel like a bonus, but when it happens and it's not as a result of using hormonal contraception, it can be due to a potentially harmful cause. It's easy to assume fewer or absent periods are perimenopause, but it can be a sign of the body being energy deficient. There's a risk of being misdiagnosed with perimenopause when in fact you have relative energy deficiency in sport (REDs), which has the potential to cause long-term harm to your body, including to your bone health (see chapter 16).

When to see your doctor

You have enough to cope with in perimenopause without heavy bleeding limiting your lifestyle too. There are lots of things that can be tried. Remember that a change in your bleeding can indicate underlying conditions that need treatment or monitoring. See your doctor if:

- Your periods are heavy and affecting your ability to live your daily life.
- You're bleeding in between your periods.
- You're bleeding after sex.
- You have any vaginal bleeding at all when you are in post-menopause – it's very important to rule out endometrial cancer.
- Bleeding persists for three to six months after starting on HRT.
- You've been stable on HRT for six months and you have unexpected bleeding.
- Your period pain is significant and not eased by simple painkillers.
- You have any unusual, discoloured or smelly vaginal discharge.
- You are concerned you may have a sexually transmitted infection.
- You feel excessively tired, faint or look pale.
- You are bleeding from other areas such as your gums or anus, or there is blood in your urine.

WHEN YOU CAN'T RUN

Sometimes a heavy or painful period makes you feel unable to run. It can be worth giving it a go and seeing how you feel. You might be surprised, but sometimes it's just out of the question. Try to focus on what you can do rather than what you can't. Could you go for a walk, try some gentle yoga or do some stretching? Alternatively, pull the duvet over your head and don't give exercise another thought. This is definitely a time for self-compassion.

CHAPTER 7

Breasts

Breasts are no less relevant or important when you reach menopause. In fact, it's a crucial time for us to pay them extra attention. Breasts are very sensitive to hormonal changes, so problems often arise during perimenopause. As well as trying to overcome these in order to run, we need to be thinking about creating good lifestyle habits to reduce our risk of breast cancer, which increases as we get older.

BREAST CHANGES DURING MENOPAUSE

Even if you've never struggled with breast problems before, there are a number of changes and symptoms that you might experience in menopause. These include:

- Breast tenderness.
- Breast pain.
- Change in breast size and consistency.
- Sagging of breasts.
- Skin changes.

Look at page 59 for a reminder of the structure of the breast, because it's helpful to understand what's going on and why you might be getting issues.

Breast pain and tenderness

More than half of women experience breast pain, also known as mastalgia, at some point in their lives. Two-thirds of breast pain is

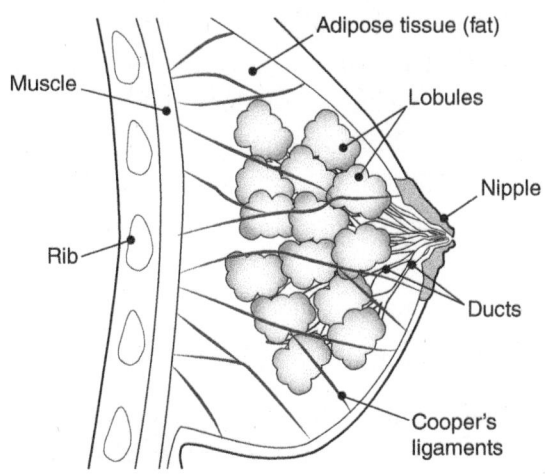

Internal structure of the breast

cyclical, which means the pain is linked to the menstrual cycle and happens at the same stage of the cycle each month, usually just before a period starts. The remaining third is non-cyclical pain, which doesn't have a link to menstruation and can happen at any time for any number of days. A survey done at the London Marathon in 2012 found that 32 per cent of the 1285 female runners surveyed experienced mastalgia and 17 per cent of them said that their breast pain affected their exercise habits.

Cyclical pain

Breast tissues are affected by the changing hormone levels of the menstrual cycle. Oestrogen and progesterone levels rise each month and trigger changes to prepare the body for a potential pregnancy. Blood supply to the breasts increases, and milk ducts and lobules start enlarging. This can make your breasts feel swollen, tight and sore, and they might feel lumpy, too. The very idea of running and intentionally jiggling your breasts up and down is laughable.

Cyclical pain tends to be generalised in both breasts, most commonly in the upper outer part with some spreading into the top of the arms and armpits. Premenstrual breast pain usually eases once your period starts. During perimenopause, you may get more frequent periods, which can mean you're struggling with breast pain more often. If you develop bigger gaps between your bleeds, you might spend longer with that premenstrual feeling or the symptoms might feel more intense.

Non-cyclical pain

Breast pain not linked to periods is also very common and, of course, as you move into late perimenopause and post-menopause, when you're no longer having cycles, it becomes more relevant. It tends to be more localised to one area of one breast as opposed to the more diffuse pattern of cyclical pain.

Non-cyclical pain clears on its own in around half of women, but there's sometimes an underlying cause such as:

- Infection or inflammation of the breast tissue (mastitis).
- Injury – a knock to the breast can hurt for some time afterwards.
- Breast cyst.
- Breast abscess.
- Benign (non-cancerous) tumours of the breast.
- Breast cancer – very unlikely to be the main and only symptom.
- Side-effect of medications, including some antidepressants and hormonal treatments.
- Previous breast surgery.

Sometimes the pain isn't coming from the breast tissue itself, but from the structures around it, such as the muscle, cartilage or ribs, which are behind the breast, and from the nerves that supply these structures. The pain could even originate from the lungs, heart or gall bladder.

GOOD TO KNOW

Around 50 per cent of women say their breasts hurt when they exercise. When there are no other breast problems, this is called exercise-induced breast pain. Not surprisingly, the bigger your breasts are and the more vigorous and bounce-inducing the activity, the more likely you are to get pain.

A study done by the University of Portsmouth showed that breast pain is more common in women who are not fit and active. They point out that this could be because people who don't have breast pain might be able to exercise more, rather than the possibility that increased levels of exercise result in reduced breast pain.

TREATMENTS FOR BREAST PAIN

Many women just put up with breast pain or haven't found ways to ease it. The most relief seems to come from a very supportive bra that minimises breast movement. Wearing two bras or a tight-fitting crop top over a bra is a trick some runners use to reduce bounce, and the front straps on running backpacks can help too. A padded bra can feel most comfortable if your breasts are very sensitive and try wearing a soft bra at night if breast pain is stopping you sleeping. Simple painkillers such as paracetamol, ibuprofen or topical (applied to the skin) diclofenac may relieve pain and make running more comfortable. Hot or cold compresses can ease discomfort, too.

There are a range of lifestyle measures recommended, such as eating a low-fat diet, reducing caffeine or adding flaxseeds to your food. The evidence for them is limited, but they aren't going to harm you so you might want to explore them. Similarly, evening primrose oil, vitamin B6 and vitamin E supplements don't have enough evidence to recommend them to all women, but anecdotally some women find they help.

For really severe cases there are some heavy-duty hormonal treatments which specialists sometimes prescribe, but they can have significant side-effects, so a careful discussion with your doctor about the risks and benefits is needed.

> ## GOOD TO KNOW
>
> It's common to experience breast pain when you're using HRT, especially when you first start taking it or after a dose change. Breast tissue can be affected by both the progestogen and oestrogen in hormone therapy. Thankfully it usually settles down within a few months.

> ### When to see your doctor
>
> Get to know your breasts really well so you can spot any changes. See your doctor if:
>
> - You have cyclical breast pain of more than three months that is severe, isn't improving with self-help measures and is affecting your quality of life.
> - You have non-cyclical pain that isn't resolving after a couple of weeks or is getting increasingly severe.
> - You generally have concerns about your breast pain.
> - You notice any changes in your breast or nipple that are not normal for you. This might be a lump, skin change or shape irregularity. Whatever it is, get it checked.

STRUCTURAL BREAST CHANGES

Aside from breast pain and tenderness, you might notice changes in the size and position of your breasts as you move through peri- and into post-menopause.

Breasts are largely made up of adipose (fatty) tissue, so if you gain body fat in perimenopause, they might get bigger. More commonly, though, women say that their breasts get smaller and feel empty, especially towards and during post-menopause. Breast lobes and lobules, previously used for milk production, shrink, which makes breasts feel less dense and have a smaller volume.

If your nipples are heading south and your breasts are sitting lower on your chest, be reassured this isn't due to your running. It's thanks to a combination of gravity, changes in your skin and reduced breast volume. The skin overlying your breasts is one of the main support mechanisms for your breast tissue. As we move through menopause our skin becomes less elastic, doesn't have the rebound and strength it used to, and is less able to keep breasts pert and high. Breast tissue is also supported by Cooper's ligaments, which run throughout the breast. Like all connective tissues, they lose some of their collagen content with age and become less effective at supporting the breast. Breast ptosis is the medical term for sagging breasts and the biggest factor determining how much ptosis you will get is your genetics, and not how far you run.

> 'I've suffered with very sore breasts during perimenopause, but it's never hindered my running, I think because I'm barely an A cup, so there isn't much to jig about!'
> **Sarah**

SPORTS BRAS AND MENOPAUSE

Around 70 per cent of women are wearing the wrong size bra. The chest band is usually too big and the cup too small. Nothing replaces going to a shop with a wide range of sports bras and a highly trained fitter to get the right bra for you. You need to lose your inhibitions and jog and jump around in front of the mirror to see how much your breasts move. Don't assume you know what bra size you need, because the fit is the most important thing.

A lot has been learned from extensive studies done by the Research Group for Breast Health (RGBH) at the University of Portsmouth. Breasts move in a figure of eight pattern when you run, but the bulk of the movement is in a vertical direction. There's more sideways movement in agility sports. Finding the right bra isn't always easy and there are some important points you need to consider when it comes to sports bras during menopause:

- Your breasts will change and you may need to have multiple bra fits as you move from peri- to post-menopause. You may also need to have sports bras of different sizes if your breasts change a lot throughout your cycle.
- The way your breasts move when you run changes. Breast tissue becomes less elastic as you get older and studies have shown that older women's breasts move less than younger women's. This might be good news if you're someone who experiences exercise-induced breast pain. It can also mean that you have a wider choice of sports bras that will keep you bounce-free. You still need optimum support, though.
- Your bra might start to rub when it hasn't before. Skin can become drier, thinner and more sensitive around menopause. In addition, you might be sweating more than you used to when you run. An optimal bra fit and applying lubricant to your skin before you run can help. Look for wide and padded straps if the chafing is on your shoulders. For more about skin changes in menopause, see chapter 13.

You deserve a good sports bra, even if your breasts feel in some way redundant or you think all hope of pertness is lost forever. The right bra will ensure you're comfortable and will help to make you an efficient runner. Don't give up on your breasts. You also need to be super-aware of how your breasts look and feel, so you can spot any changes that might indicate breast disease.

BREAST CANCER

It's not menopause itself which increases our risk of breast cancer, it's getting older that's to blame. Around 75 per cent of breast cancer cases are in women over 50 years of age. I can't do justice to the topic here and I recommend reading *The Complete Guide to Breast Cancer* by Professor Trisha Greenhalgh and Dr Liz O'Riordan, both doctors with first-hand experience of breast cancer. I want to focus on how running can help and why it's worth overcoming barriers that prevent you from running.

Being active is a crucial part of preventing breast cancer, managing it if you do have it and reducing the risk of it returning. In fact, exercising regularly can reduce your risk of breast cancer occurring or coming back by 30 per cent. This is a huge percentage. It's not fully understood exactly how exercise reduces the risk. Some of its effect may be through lowering body-fat levels. Women who are obese have a higher risk of breast cancer than those who are not. Higher levels of visceral fat (see chapter 12) result in increased inflammation in the body and more resistance to insulin, both of which can increase breast cancer risk. Oestrogen is made in fat cells and higher levels of oestrogen can lead to an increased risk of breast cancer in some women. Using exercise, both aerobic and strength exercise, to reduce body-fat levels could therefore be one of the mechanisms by which exercise lowers risk.

Exercise improves and activates our immune system, including causing the release of natural killer cells which recognise cancer cells as abnormal and try to destroy them. In addition, exercise itself is thought to be anti-inflammatory, not just through reducing visceral fat levels, but also through the release of anti-inflammatory substances called myokines, which are released from our muscles when we're active. Reducing chronic (long-term) inflammation reduces the risk of many medical conditions, including cancer.

If you're diagnosed with breast cancer, then regular exercise, and that includes running, is a very important part of your treatment plan. Not only will it help you to feel fit for the treatment, but it can help to minimise the side-effects, including those of fatigue and anxiety. It gives you something that you can control, helps you to trust your body and to keep your identity.

There is still a lot we don't understand, but the message is clear – all movement is good. Of course, breast cancer still happens to women who are regular runners and there are many factors that cause it. I'm not pretending that running prevents all breast cancer, but it is one very positive and powerful thing we can all do for our breast health now and into the future.

> 'It was a great relief when everything had settled down after my breast surgery and I could put my trainers on, get out the door, be free and be me again. No one checking how I was or not knowing what to say. Just cheery smiles as I ran past.'
> **Anonymous**

LOOKING AFTER YOUR BREASTS

My take-home message is that being breast aware is more important than it's ever been for us in our pre-menopausal days. Here are some simple things you can do that could save your life:

1. Get into the habit of checking your breasts. Get to know how they feel, so you can spot any changes. Set a reminder on your calendar, such as the first day of every month, to make it easy.
2. Attend breast screening appointments. A short-lived discomfort is worth it for reassurance or early detection of something that needs treating.
3. Keep running, but make sure you do strength work too. Both are needed to give you the most protection against breast cancer happening or recurring and to get maximum benefit during any treatment.
4. Address lifestyle factors. Reduce your alcohol intake to lower risk and eat a varied, nutritious diet to help you maintain a healthy weight. Smoking is now thought to contribute to breast cancer.
5. Only a small number of breast cancers are linked to inherited faulty genes. If you have a family history of breast, ovarian or other related cancers, then speak to your doctor about whether genetic testing might be appropriate. It depends on the number of family members, their relation to you and their ages when they were diagnosed.

GOOD TO KNOW

There are many myths to dispel. Despite what you may read in your social media feeds, the following will not cause breast cancer:

- Carrying your mobile phone in your bra while you run or just go about daily life.
- Using antiperspirants and deodorants to stop sweating during exercise.
- Wearing an underwired bra.
- Getting a knock or injury to your breast.
- Having pierced nipples.
- Being exposed to chemicals in your everyday environment, such as in the air, on foods or in plastic.

CHAPTER 8

Bladders and Bits

Genitourinary syndrome of menopause (GSM) is a new term created to acknowledge the range of urinary and vaginal symptoms that women can experience. Problems begin in perimenopause and over half of women in post-menopause are affected by GSM. There are oestrogen and progesterone receptors in the bladder, urethra (tube from the bladder to the outside) and pelvic floor, so it's easy to see why the falling levels of these hormones directly affect the structure and function of the urinary tract, as well as the supporting tissues around them, including those of the vagina and vulva.

Here are some of the problems you might experience with GSM:

- Needing to pee more often.
- Needing to pee during the night.
- An urgency to get to the toilet.
- Leaking urine.
- Urine not flowing as strongly.
- Frequent urinary tract infections.
- Vaginal dryness.
- Vaginal and vulval itch.
- Vaginal irritation and burning.
- Painful sex (dyspareunia).

Bladder symptoms are a major issue for runners: needing to be near a toilet restricts how far you can run and fear of leaking urine means many women don't run at all. Vulval and vaginal symptoms can make running uncomfortable. Unlike most other menopause symptoms, these problems don't get better on their own. In fact, they usually get worse over time, so they need treatment, but around 70 per cent of women with GSM don't seek help. These symptoms can hugely affect self-esteem and quality of life, and we shouldn't accept that this is all a natural part of ageing. I'm very grateful to pelvic health physiotherapist Emma Brockwell for her guidance and input to this chapter.

> ## GOOD TO KNOW
>
> The pelvic floor is a sling of muscles which attach to your pubic bone at the front and your coccyx at the back. They work together to support your bladder, uterus and bowel, which sit on top of the muscular sling. The pelvic floor muscles contain both slow-twitch (70 per cent) and fast-twitch (30 per cent) muscle fibres. The slow-twitch fibres offer continuous support and keep urine in the bladder until you reach a toilet. The fast-twitch fibres activate to stop urine leaking out when you laugh or sneeze. When you do pelvic floor exercises, it's important to exercise both types of fibre with both long and short squeezes.

BLADDER FUNCTION

Declining oestrogen levels in menopause directly affect the stability and strength of both the pelvic floor muscles, which support the bladder, and the muscular wall of the bladder. Weaker and less stable muscles mean reduced bladder support, urine leaks and more frequent bladder contractions. There is a triangular area at the base of the bladder called the trigone. One of its roles is to detect bladder fullness, and stretch receptors in the trigone send messages to the brain that you need to pass urine. Most of the oestrogen receptors in the bladder are in the trigone and it's thought that oestrogen helps to keep this area thick and elastic. When oestrogen levels are low, the trigone can become thin and not stretch as it should, resulting in poor bladder function.

The tissues of the urethra, which takes urine from the bladder to the outside, also become thinner and less elastic with oestrogen decline. This makes them less able to sustain pressure and stop urine leaking out. Collagen provides the structure and scaffold of connective tissues, and oestrogen affects collagen synthesis. It's likely that menopause and age-related reduction of collagen reduces the supportiveness of the tissues around the bladder and urethra.

There are oestrogen receptors in the brain and the message to start peeing comes from the brain, but it's not yet known what effect oestrogen levels have on bladder control via this pathway.

Overactive bladders (OAB)

The average person passes urine six or seven times in 24 hours. You'll often hear menopausal women say they have a 'small bladder' and that is certainly how it can feel. In reality, the bladder is probably of normal size, it's just that the muscular wall contracts more frequently than it should. This is called an overactive bladder (OAB). There are a number of factors that cause OAB and it's usually a combination of several of the following:

- Low oestrogen levels which affect bladder function.
- Concentrated urine which irritates the bladder wall.
- Bladder irritants such as caffeine and alcohol.
- Constipation where bulky faeces press on the bladder and obstruct the flow of urine.
- Urine infections which commonly irritate the bladder.
- An overactive pelvic floor which doesn't allow the bladder to fill and empty properly.
- Other medical conditions, such as diabetes, bladder tumours and neurological conditions.

Treatment for overactive bladders

OAB can be difficult to manage as a runner. You're juggling trying not to drink too much before a run, planning routes with toilets and timing race portaloo visits. There are things that might help. Firstly, don't restrict your fluid intake, and avoid caffeine and alcohol to minimise bladder irritation. Sometimes the sensation to pee isn't genuine, so stay calm, especially before a race. Try to distract yourself and relax. This can progress to bladder training, which is best done with professional guidance, but gradually leaving longer and longer between toilet visits, aiming for four hours, can build your confidence and reprogramme your bladder. Don't forget the possibility of an underlying cause and it's best to see your GP before you self-treat.

There are medications that can help OAB, including bladder relaxant tablets. These can be effective, but do have side-effects. Vaginal oestrogens can help stall or reverse the thinning of vaginal tissues, which may help bladder symptoms. Your GP can refer you to a women's health physiotherapist or urologist who may use other treatments, including transcutaneous or percutaneous tibial nerve stimulation (TTNS or PTNS), where electrical impulses are sent to the posterior tibial nerve, at the ankle, which is a nerve that contributes to bladder control. Electrical impulses can also be sent to the bladder muscles via vaginal or anal probes. Bladder botox may be available in some regions and, finally, there are surgical options for extreme cases.

Stress urinary incontinence

With OAB you might leak urine if you don't get to the toilet in time. This is called urge incontinence, but there is another type of incontinence called stress urinary incontinence (SUI). This is when you leak urine when you cough, sneeze or jump. This affects at least one in three women and is more common after menopause. In fact, over the age of 50, half of women are affected. Incontinence can be a mixture of stress and urge incontinence.

Although SUI is common, it is not a normal part of ageing and we shouldn't just put up with it, because help and treatment are available. SUI is a huge barrier to women being active, particularly to high-impact exercise, such as running. This is so sad, as we know vigorous exercise improves cardiovascular health and high-impact activity strengthens bones. Not being able to do this due to SUI is harming the long-term health of women.

> 'I've put up with leaking urine for years. It's not too bad in winter, black leggings can hide a lot of urine, but I really want to be able to wear flimsy shorts on long, hot summer runs. I know I need to get over my embarrassment and get some help.'
> **Anonymous**

The mechanics of stress incontinence

Your bladder expands as it fills with urine. The bladder neck and urethra are kept closed by the pelvic floor muscles and surrounding tissues. Normally you choose when to relax these and let urine out. If the pelvic floor muscles are weak or if the pressure on the pelvic floor is too much, then the muscles can't cope and urine leaks out unintentionally. There are a number of things that can increase the pressure inside the pelvis and weaken the pelvic floor muscles. These include:

- Being pregnant.
- Giving birth, particularly if baby was big or the delivery was difficult.
- Low oestrogen levels.
- Constipation.
- Recurrent coughing.
- Heavy lifting.
- Being overweight.

Running is a repetitive, high-impact exercise and tests the pelvic floor. When you land, the pressure inside the pelvis increases and over long periods of time this can weaken the pelvic floor muscles. Running can certainly reveal stress incontinence and during peri- or post-menopause is when it's most likely to appear.

Treatment for stress incontinence

I don't want you to wear an incontinence pad, always wear black running tights or avoid drinking before you run. And I definitely don't want you to stop running. I want you to go and see a women's health physiotherapist. These are professionals who are specifically trained to treat women with urinary incontinence. More than 60 per cent of women find the treatment successful. Your GP can refer you to a women's health physiotherapist or you can visit one privately. In the UK you can use the search tool on the Pelvic Obstetric and Gynaecological Physiotherapy (POGP) website to find one near you (thepogp.co.uk).

You can start pelvic floor exercises (Kegels) right away and get the neural pathways to those muscles activated, but you need more than this. Leaking urine is a symptom of pelvic floor dysfunction and you need a thorough assessment of your pelvic floor, your posture and biomechanics. Sometimes pelvic floor muscles are weak because they are overactive and don't relax properly. Sometimes weaknesses or imbalances in the muscles around your pelvis, such as your glutes, contribute to stress incontinence. Your running form and gait may be adding to the pressure on your pelvic floor, too. You will be given a treatment plan that is far more than just a few pelvic floor squeezes and you may have to reduce or temporarily stop your running while having treatment. It's boring, it's hard work and it can take months, but it will be worth it. Treatments can involve:

- Pelvic floor exercises.
- Vaginal exercisers and weights.
- Electrical stimulation of the muscles.
- Strength and conditioning exercises for the core, glutes, hip and leg muscles.
- Posture correction.
- Breathing exercises.
- Running gait advice, including taking shorter strides and landing on your midfoot rather than your heel.

GOOD TO KNOW

Normal pelvic floor functioning is dependent on good breathing. Check in with your breathing from time to time and see what it's like. Some women are breath-holders or take very shallow breaths, particularly at times of stress. When you fill your lungs, breathe deeply and blow your belly out as you do so. Your pelvic floor muscles should relax as you do this. When you're breathing out is when the pressure in the abdomen and pelvis reduces, and the pelvic floor muscles contract and rise. Practise this breathing technique multiple times a day to reprogramme your breathing.

PELVIC ORGAN PROLAPSE

Another consequence of increased pelvic pressure and weak pelvic floor muscles is a prolapse. Your bladder, uterus and bowel sit on your pelvic floor hammock, but can bulge through and give you the sensation of heaviness, dragging or 'something coming down'. You might feel a swelling or lump in your vagina. Gravity is an exacerbating factor, so this can start after a long run or when you've been on your feet for hours. If it's your bladder that's prolapsing, it's called a cystocele and you'll get urinary symptoms such as urge and stress incontinence, not being able to empty your bladder properly and urinary frequency. If your bowel is dropping down, it's called a rectocele and you can get constipated, and find it difficult to empty your bowel or wipe your bottom clean. You might also get faecal urgency or incontinence. When the uterus drops, it's called a uterine prolapse. Sex can be uncomfortable or painful with any type of prolapse.

Treatment for a prolapse

There are different degrees of prolapse, from very mild to very severe. The degree determines the treatment and also whether or not you need to stop running. If you're advised to stop running, follow the advice, because this will be the quickest way to return to running. Again, a women's health physiotherapist is who you need to see, but your GP may refer you straight to a gynaecologist for more severe prolapses. Here are some tips if you have a pelvic organ prolapse:

- Do daily, good quality pelvic floor exercises.
- Avoid heavy lifting until you've been guided how to do so correctly by a physio.
- Lose excess weight.
- Avoid constipation at all costs – drink plenty of fluid, and have a diet full of fruit and vegetables.
- See your doctor for treatment of any persistent cough.
- Avoid holding your breath during exercise.
- Avoid sitting on the toilet for a long time.

- Open your bowels in a squat position – put your feet up on a step (or pile of books) and lean forward a little.

Pessaries are plastic devices that can be very helpful for controlling a prolapse. They come in many different shapes, but the ring pessary is the most common. They're inserted into the vagina, where they act as a support to hold everything up. You will usually be prescribed some vaginal oestrogen to use alongside, to make sure the vaginal tissues stay healthy. If conservative measures don't work, surgery is also an option and there are many different surgical techniques. Whichever option you choose, continue following the tips on the previous page.

> 'After prolapse surgery I felt like I needed more guidance and went to a private physio, who has been amazing. I'm running long distances now and doing strength work. I wish I'd been better informed before I had surgery, so that I knew what was coming, but also so I knew it was going to be okay.'
>
> **Colette,** Lancaster

ATROPHIC VAGINITIS

Changes to the vagina and vulva are part of GSM and affect around half of post-menopausal women. The terms vaginal atrophy, atrophic vaginitis and vulvovaginal atrophy are all used to describe these changes. Healthy vaginal tissue has a good blood supply and is thick, rippled, elastic and moist. It's also slightly acidic with a great population of lactobacilli bacteria to prevent infections, and plenty of vaginal mucous to act as lubrication and to keep out germs. There are lots of oestrogen receptors in the vagina, especially in the lining. When oestrogen levels fall, over time the vaginal lining becomes flatter, thinner, drier and less elastic. This is vaginal atrophy. The number of lactobacilli decreases, too. The tissues can become inflamed. This is vaginitis. These changes lead to a number of symptoms including:

- Painful sex.
- Discomfort during cervical screening.
- Vaginal dryness, itch and burning.
- Urinary frequency.
- Dysuria – burning when you wee.
- Vaginal infections.
- Urinary infections.
- Spotting of blood (never assume atrophic vaginitis is the cause).
- Discomfort from long runs.
- Pain sitting on a bike saddle.

Treatments for atrophic vaginitis

As runners, we get extra sweaty and take a lot of showers. Over-washing and using perfumed products can strip away our natural body oils and healthy bacteria, and upset the pH of our genitals. This can make vaginal and urinary infections more likely and irritate the delicate atrophic tissues. Avoid washing too much and just use plain water. Steer clear of douching. Your vagina is self-cleaning. It doesn't need feminine hygiene washes and it certainly doesn't need steaming.

You can ease the symptoms of atrophic vaginitis with a vaginal moisturiser. You can buy these over the counter. Look for ones which are fragrance free. If long runs are uncomfortable, use it before you run. If your symptoms are mainly at the labia (lips) rather than further inside, a smear of Vaseline might be enough to stop chafing. Regular sex helps to keep your vagina healthy, but if sex is uncomfortable use a water-based lubricant.

Finally, rather than just soothing dryness, you can treat the cause by replacing oestrogen. Because there are so many oestrogen receptors in the vaginal lining, a good option is to use a vaginal oestrogen which works directly on the local tissues. Systemic (full body) HRT can help, too. For more about these options, see chapter 15.

New vaginal symptoms should always be checked by your doctor or nurse. Itch, discharge and skin changes can be the result of more than just atrophic vaginitis, and vaginal infections need to be ruled out.

> 'After long marathon-training runs I was crying when the shower water hurt me, avoiding going to the toilet, and lying on the sofa because it was so painful to sit. I discovered Juliet's blog about vaginal atrophy and cried with relief. Vaginal oestrogen and HRT have been a game-changer. It's the difference between me running and not, having a sex life and better bladder control. I feel great and I'm running another marathon. Don't suffer in silence or think this will go away. Listen to your body and get help.'
> **Ruth Forrest**

URINARY TRACT INFECTIONS

Many menopausal women are plagued by urinary tract infections (UTIs). The menopausal changes in the urethra, vagina and vulval tissues mean there is a reduced defence to germs. UTIs can be in the bladder with short bouts of cystitis, but can also extend to the kidneys where deeper infections can make you very unwell.

It's usually pretty obvious when you have a UTI. You might have low abdominal pain, keep needing to go for a wee, and experience stinging and burning in your bladder and urethra when you do. UTIs are grim. Sometimes there is just some inflammation in the bladder and a few days of paracetamol, drinking plenty and rest will be enough to clear things. You can also try products which alter the pH of the urine and make it less acidic, such as cranberry juice and sachets of potassium citrate from the pharmacy. There's debate as to how effective they are, but they may give some relief.

If infection takes hold, you may have a temperature, feel nauseated and pass blood in your urine (haematuria). You may need to see a doctor as you could need antibiotics if bacteria are grown from your urine sample (see the box on page 78).

Occasionally UTIs are subtler and they just upset normal bladder function, giving symptoms of OAB or SUI. If you're getting frequent UTIs in menopause, go back to the basics of looking after your vulval and vaginal tissues by avoiding irritants and replacing oestrogen. Always pee after sex. Increasing fluid intake can make a big difference, too. As runners, we're at risk of dehydration and as menopausal women we might not feel thirst in the same way as we used to due to thirst sensations altering with age and possibly hormonal fluctuations. We might also be losing extra fluid through hot sweats. Make sure you drink before, during and after your run and throughout the day, too. Remember that staying well and having a good immune system involves your wider health, so balancing your training, fuelling and stress levels are important. Recurrent UTIs might need further investigations to rule out other causes and your doctor will refer you on if needed.

When to see your doctor

Your doctor can determine the likely cause of your urinary symptoms, start treatments and if necessary refer you on for further treatment, investigation and opinions. It's always a good idea to take a sample of urine with you. Take a mid-stream sample (let the first bit go into the toilet) in a sterile pot. A bladder diary noting when and how much you wee or leak is helpful, too. You can download one from various websites, including Bladder and Bowel UK (bbuk.org.uk). See your doctor if:

- You leak urine.
- You have an overactive bladder that is affecting your daily life.
- You think you have a urine infection and over-the-counter treatment hasn't helped after three days, or you have a high temperature, vomiting or low back pain.
- You have recurrent urine infections.
- There is any blood in your urine.
- You're passing more urine than normal and feel tired, thirsty or are losing weight.
- You have symptoms of vulval or vaginal atrophy.
- You think you have a prolapse.

CHAPTER 9

Bowels

Bowels are a very important topic for runners generally, and there are a number of changes that women experience around menopause that can impact training. These might be new and unexpected or a flare-up of pre-existing bowel issues. Either way, it can be a tricky time and take a bit of trial and error to get things right. There are also other bowel-related health problems that crop up around this time of our lives.

BOWEL CANCER

Let's start with the most important message: don't assume a change in your bowel habit is down to menopause. If your bowels have been behaving differently for three weeks or more, you should see your doctor. The changes that are important are:

- Abdominal or bottom pain.
- New diarrhoea (without an obvious cause).
- New constipation.
- A mixture of diarrhoea and constipation.
- Blood in your poo.
- Feeling you haven't fully emptied your bowels.
- Feeling very tired or losing weight unexpectedly.

These symptoms don't mean you have bowel cancer, but you may need tests to rule it out. Bowel cancer risk increases as we get older and the charity Bowel Cancer UK states that more than nine out of 10 new cases are diagnosed in people over 50. It's the third most common cancer in women in the UK, after breast and lung, and one in 20 women will get bowel cancer during their lifetime. The earlier it's picked up, the easier it is to treat and the better the chances of cure and survival.

Remember, regular running helps to reduce your risk of bowel cancer by as much as 25 to 50 per cent. That's a huge reduction and this is thanks to a number of factors, including reducing constipation, meaning any carcinogens (cancer-forming substances) in poo have a shorter contact time with the bowel wall, lowering inflammation in the body generally and the activation of natural killer cells, which may help fight bowel cancer. If you're already running regularly when you're diagnosed with bowel cancer, your chances of survival are greater than someone who is inactive. After being treated for bowel cancer, exercising regularly can help to reduce the risk of recurrence by around 40 per cent. These are all reasons we should be more active at this time of life rather than follow the accepted route of becoming less active as we age.

THE GUT MICROBIOME

The gut microbiome is the community of trillions of microorganisms living in our digestive system, mostly in the large intestine. It includes bacteria, viruses, fungi and parasites, the exact combination of which is individual to each of us. It's only in recent years that the importance of having a healthy gut microbiome has come to light and we still don't fully understand the extent of its roles.

The gut microbiome helps with digestion of food and smooth transit of faeces, but its impact goes well beyond the gut. It communicates with multiple body systems via chemical messages. For example, in addition to being made in the brain, melatonin and serotonin are also made in the gut, and the production of these and the response of the brain can be impacted by gut microbes. These hormones are crucial in regulating mood and sleep, and some people who sleep poorly have been found to have restricted rather than diverse gut microbes. The microbes are also thought to break down chemicals which are harmful to sleep. In addition to our digestive and mental health, gut microbes also have an effect on our immune, nervous and endocrine systems.

We don't fully understand the effects of menopause on the gut microbiome. Research is patchy, but suggests that high levels of circulating oestrogen and progesterone help maintain a diverse range of gut microbes. Some studies have shown the microbiome of post-menopausal women is less diverse than pre-menopausal women and it changes to resemble that of men. The health impact of that change is unknown. It could be protective, harmful or a mixture of both. The microbiome may also affect the amount of hormones in the blood. One of the theories is that gut microbes can grab oestrogen that's been processed in the liver and is ready to be excreted in faeces, and put it back into the circulation.

The gut microbiome seems to have a role in the regulation of bone metabolism and the development of, and possibly treatment of, osteoporosis. More research needs to be done before we can draw any definite conclusions, including what effect HRT has on the gut microbiome, and whether the microbiome itself has any influence over when menopause actually occurs and the severity of symptoms.

What we do know is that trying to establish and maintain a healthy and diverse gut microbiome is a positive thing to do. While a good diet is essential (for more about gut microbiome-friendly foods, see chapter 16), it's important to know that your genetics, environment and lifestyle all have an influence, too. Antibiotic use, lack of sleep, not eating enough and high stress can all damage the gut microbiome.

Running can support a healthy gut microbiome. Studies have shown that moderate- to high-intensity exercise such as running has the biggest impact on microorganism diversity and abundance, more so than resistance exercise. The most consistent changes were seen in people who did moderate- to high-intensity, but especially high-intensity, aerobic exercise for more than 30 minutes, three or more times a week, for more than eight weeks. Not only can exercise increase the 'good bacteria', but it can reduce the 'bad bacteria', too. This is undoubtedly one of the ways that running improves health. This is an exciting area of research and there is much more to learn.

> ### GOOD TO KNOW
> Don't waste your money on over-the-counter or internet tests which check the health of your gut microbiome and often try to sell you expensive supplements afterwards. These are not recommended, because not enough is known about what numbers and types of microorganisms reflect a good microbiome in individual people, and how they affect your health. The results aren't helpful.

CONSTIPATION

The hormonal changes of menopause slow down the speed that food travels through the gut, so there's more time for water to be reabsorbed and stools to become harder. Being constipated is uncomfortable, can give you belly ache, bloating and make you feel nauseated. More importantly, it can have an effect on your wider health. Constipation can increase the risk of bowel cancer and harm the gut microbiome. Sitting on the loo for prolonged periods of time, straining when you open your bowels and having a load of poo stuck inside you can increase your risk of developing piles (haemorrhoids) and weaken your pelvic floor muscles, putting you at an increased risk of stress urinary incontinence and pelvic organ prolapse.

The number one step to avoid constipation is to drink enough fluid, although we tend to get less thirsty in menopause. Increasing your fluid intake throughout the day, and especially after running to account for fluid lost in flushes, sweats and exercise, can make a big difference. A top tip is to drink a glass of water first thing in the morning. Keep a large water bottle in the fridge and try to make sure it's empty by the end of the day. Remember that all fluids count so if you don't like plain water, then drink well-diluted cordials or herbal teas instead. Next, increase your fibre intake. For more on what to put in your shopping basket, see chapter 16, but essentially lots of fruit and vegetables, and other high-fibre foods, will help stools pass smoothly through your gut. The more fibre you eat, the more fluid you need to drink. Otherwise you'll end up constipated. Finally, remember that movement is one of the most effective tools to avoid constipation. Running is a perfect way to regulate your bowel habit, but you need to avoid being too sedentary and move regularly through the day, too. You might find you're getting more constipated if you're running less due to menopause symptoms.

> 'I've definitely found I'm more bloated in menopause. I do get constipated sometimes, so I'm really trying to eat more fibre and I know I don't drink nearly enough water.'
> **Kate**

GOOD TO KNOW

Menopause does not cause irritable bowel syndrome (IBS) but you may be diagnosed with it while you are in menopause and, if you already have it, it may get worse for a while. Fluctuations in hormone levels and extra stress in life can cause flare-ups of IBS, which includes symptoms such as constipation, diarrhoea, bloating and abdominal pain. Managing IBS is an ongoing challenge for those that have it. Lifestyle is key and help from a dietician can be invaluable. Guts UK (gutscharity.org.uk) will put you on the right track.

DIARRHOEA

You might experience some loose stools in menopause, but don't forget, if you have a change in your bowel habit that lasts three weeks or more, you need to see your doctor.

High stress can increase the speed at which food moves through the gut and some women also find that their gut becomes more sensitive in menopause. There may be certain foods that you no longer seem to be able to tolerate. These are usually temporary intolerances not food allergies.

With a more sensitive bowel, you might develop the runner's trots or, if you already struggle with it, find it becomes more severe. This is the sudden urge to open your bowels triggered by the action of running. The jiggling around of the bowel and the adrenalin released when you run speeds up the time it takes for food to move through the bowel. The stools are usually loose and often explosive. Spotting triggers and using trial and error is the best option. Try to be open-minded and remember that your body is changing, and you need to learn how to adapt. Here are some things you can try for runner's trots:

- **Plan your eating**: Running fasted may not suit some menopausal women (see chapter 16), so it can be a juggling act to work out how close to running you can manage to eat. Avoid running too close to a main meal and make use of small snacks around an hour before. Chew your food properly and don't rush.
- **Choose your foods**: A food diary can help you identify trigger foods. Look at what you ate the day before as well as the day of running.
- **Take care with drinks**: Caffeine stimulates the bowel, so consider ditching your pre-run coffee. Alcohol and fruit juices can upset the bowel too.
- **Warm up**: Going straight into full-on exercise can be a shock to the bowel, so wake it up gradually with an extended warm-up.
- **Train your gut**: Make changes to your training plans and schedules incrementally. Like your muscles, your gut needs to adapt to your exercise load.
- **Pick your fuel**: Sports nutrition may no longer suit you. For more about fuelling your runs, see chapter 16.
- **Chill out**: Stress hormones are only going to make this worse. Calm pre-race nerves with distraction, music and deep breathing. Introduce some calming moments into your week.
- **Prepare**: Despite all of your efforts, sometimes the trots just happen. Always carry tissues in your running belt. Allow plenty of time for toilet queues at races and know where the toilets, or the best hedges, are on your routes.

BLOATING

Feeling bloated is common in menopause. You're either retaining wind, water or both. It can make you feel uncomfortable, enormous and put you off running. Oestrogen and progesterone have an effect on both the digestive tract and the systems that regulate fluid balance. It can be difficult to tell which is causing your bloating. Bloating from wind tends to go up and down quickly and is usually related to meals. Fluid retention can also change quite quickly, but you might notice that it's not just your abdomen that's swollen – your rings might feel tight or your fingers or ankles might swell on a very long run. It may well be a mixture of both. It can also be hard to know what's bloating and what's weight gain. Bloating tends to vary more day to day and can be uncomfortable. Weight gain is more gradual with fewer fluctuations and no pain.

It's easier to prevent bloating than to resolve it once it's there. You can't fully blame your hormones – lifestyle factors and age play an important role, too. Thankfully exercise can help. If you're too uncomfortable to run, opt for a brisk walk instead. Drink plenty of fluids throughout the day and avoid excessive amounts of salt. Smaller meals can be easier to digest, and take your time when you eat, so you aren't rushing and swallowing lots of air. Some foods such as broccoli and beans can be particularly gas-inducing and it's best to avoid fizzy drinks, too. Looking after your gut microbiome is crucial. If the bloating is very hormone driven, then HRT may ease symptoms in some women.

PILES

Also known as haemorrhoids, piles are fleshy lumps of tissue and veins which appear either just outside or inside the anus. Activities which increase the pressure in the blood vessels in your rectum can cause piles, so sitting, standing or just being on your feet for long periods of time can cause or worsen them. This includes running long distances and some runners find they first have problems when they're training for a marathon or ultramarathon. Genetics play a big role here, as do childbirth and straining on the toilet. Piles become more common in menopause, because constipation is more likely, the tissues around the anus become weaker with age, and the strength and flexibility of the rectal and anal blood vessels reduce with falling hormone levels.

Piles can ache, throb and itch, and trying to open your bowels can feel like you're pooing shards of glass. Piles can also bleed, sometimes heavily. However, never assume bleeding from your bottom is due to piles. Get checked by your doctor.

Piles usually shrink on their own, but here are some things you can do in the meantime to make things more bearable and to prevent piles in the first place:

- Drink plenty of fluids.
- Increase the fibre in your diet.
- Avoid long periods of sitting or standing still.
- Exercise regularly; although very long runs might cause or worsen piles, generally being active helps to reduce the risk of constipation.
- Use a cream from the pharmacy to soothe, shrink and reduce the itch of piles.
- Apply a barrier cream to protect piles from sweat and chafing on runs.
- Lie down for an hour and use an ice pack if piles are throbbing.
- Keep your bottom clean and dry.
- See your doctor for a diagnosis and if piles are not resolving.

Not all piles cause problems. Some small ones sit there quite happily and don't cause any bother, in which case it's fine to run. If they're swollen, painful or bleeding, you'll need some time off running while they calm down. Occasionally they're agony and you need painkillers, a lot of rest, and advice from your doctor if this is the case. There are surgical options for very problematic piles that aren't going away.

It can be pretty miserable if you've got troublesome piles, stress incontinence and perimenopausal heavy bleeding all going on at once. Honestly, this is not an easy time of life for us or our pelvis!

GOOD TO KNOW

Ovarian cancer can present with many of the symptoms mentioned in this chapter and it mostly affects women over the age of 50. Bloating, constipation, abdominal pain and tenderness are all potential symptoms of a cancer in the ovaries. Weight loss, indigestion and feeling full after only eating a small amount are common, too. The symptoms are often very vague which results in most cases of ovarian cancer being more advanced by the time the diagnosis is made. This is why it's important not to put everything down to menopause and to see a doctor when you notice new changes.

ACID REFLUX AND HEARTBURN

Acid reflux isn't a bowel issue, because it stems from your stomach, which is further up your digestive tract, but this is a good place to mention it. It's a common problem for lots of people, but can begin or worsen in menopause. Women in peri- or post-menopause are almost three times as likely to have acid reflux than pre-menopausal women.

The oesophageal sphincter is a valve where your oesophagus (tube from your mouth to your stomach) joins your stomach. It opens to let food and drink into your stomach, and closes to stop them coming back up. If acidic stomach juices do regurgitate upwards, they can inflame the lining of the oesophagus, which causes a burning sensation behind your breastbone; this is called heartburn. You might also get a bad taste in your mouth or even an irritating cough. We all get a bit of acid reflux from time to time, especially if we've overindulged, but if it's happening frequently or is severe, it's called gastro-oesophageal reflux disease (GORD).

Acid reflux can be triggered by running due to the up and down motion, especially if you eat just beforehand. There might be certain foods that trigger it – caffeine, fruit juice and tomatoes are common culprits. Some sports nutrition might flare your symptoms and acid reflux can make it hard to fuel on the go. Alcohol, smoking and being overweight are all known to be related to heartburn, as are anti-inflammatories, such as ibuprofen and aspirin. When it comes to menopause, there do seem to be other factors which lead to the onset or worsening of the condition:

- Stress levels can increase in menopause which increases stomach acid production.
- Central weight gain can exacerbate symptoms by putting extra pressure on the stomach.
- What you eat might change, especially if you're craving chocolate, spicy or fatty foods, which can trigger heartburn.
- Poor sleep is linked to increased levels of GORD – it can both cause it and be a result of it.
- Hormonal fluctuations may have a direct effect on acid production and the functioning of the oesophageal sphincter, but the exact mechanisms aren't yet understood.

> 'Acid reflux is a problem for me and I take medication. I'm trying to lose some weight, too, and batch cooking is helping me maintain a healthy diet.'
> **Kerry**

Treatment involves altering your lifestyle to prevent it happening. Try raising the head of your bed around 10 centimetres to prevent acid creeping up into the oesophagus at night. Avoid trigger foods, have smaller meals and don't eat too close to running or bedtime. Do what you can to minimise stress, maximise sleep and keep exercising regularly. There are plenty of medications available over the counter to ease the symptoms of acid reflux and to reduce the amount of acid produced. Chat to your pharmacist. They will refer you on to your doctor if necessary. So far, HRT doesn't seem to be helpful for easing acid reflux. Long term, untreated GORD can cause damage to the cells of the oesophagus, and cause ulcers and eventually even oesophageal cancer in some people, so it needs to be addressed.

When to see your doctor

Don't put off going to the doctor if you have any of the changes in the list below. Both bowel and ovarian cancer are more treatable the earlier they are diagnosed. Having any of these changes does not mean you have cancer – you probably don't, but it needs to be ruled out. Your doctor can arrange tests, many of which are very simple, to give you reassurance or refer you on to services designed to spot cancer very quickly. See your doctor if:

- A change in your bowel habit lasts for three weeks or more.
- There is blood in your poo or bleeding from your bottom.
- You feel you aren't emptying your bowel properly after you've finished on the toilet.
- You experience persistent nausea, vomiting or feel full after eating a small amount.
- You have acid reflux despite over-the-counter medications.
- Food is getting stuck in your throat.
- You have unexpected weight loss.
- Constipation is not helped by lifestyle changes.
- You suffer from frequent bloating or ongoing abdominal pains.
- You experience painful piles, or abdominal or anal lumps or bumps.
- You have uncontrolled or changing IBS symptoms.

CHAPTER 10

Bones and Joints

A recent study found that 65 per cent of women around the world suffer joint and muscle pain in menopause. This makes it the most common menopause symptom experienced by women globally. It's particularly common in Asian women, with 93 per cent of Indonesian and 96 per cent of Vietnamese women complaining of body aches.

We're led to expect and accept that getting stiffer and achier is a natural part of ageing, but not all aches and pains in menopause are simply due to getting older – they come on too quickly and severely to purely be caused by the natural ageing process. There is now a term 'musculoskeletal syndrome of menopause' to reflect new knowledge and account for the growing number of women experiencing these symptoms. Fluctuating and declining oestrogen levels almost certainly play a role here. There are oestrogen receptors in joints, muscles and bones, and even though we don't yet fully understand how it all works, it's clear that menopause directly affects our musculoskeletal system. There's a high incidence of peri- and post-menopausal musculoskeletal conditions that can completely derail runners and hugely affect training.

As runners we're used to things in our musculoskeletal system hurting! We expect and tolerate muscle burning and aching as a normal part of progressing in our fitness. It's a different story when it's happening without the trigger of hard exercise. Suddenly you're getting up from the sofa like an old woman, can barely reach down to tie your laces, and twinges and niggles are happening all the time. It can be frustrating and depressing.

The problem with musculoskeletal symptoms in menopause is that they can make us less active. The less you do, the less you can do and we begin to see a snowball effect. Any symptoms of menopause, such as mood swings, sleep or anxiety, that were being helped by activity can get worse. You begin to feel less in control, which again worsens symptoms. You can see how the snowball gets bigger and gathers momentum.

We need to remember that what we do at this point in our lives also determines our future. Our ability to live an independent life is highly dependent on how mobile we are. Continuing to move through menopause is crucial. Here are the main players in the musculoskeletal system:

- Bones – a framework of 206 bones in the adult body.
- Joints – where a bone meets a bone.
- Ligaments – run bone to bone around a joint to help to stabilise it.
- Muscles – contraction and relaxation create movement.
- Tendons – connect muscles to bones.
- Cartilage – cushions and protects bone, and is softer than bone.
- Synovial fluid – within the joint capsule.

We're going to cover bones, joints and ligaments in this chapter, and move on to muscles and tendons in the next one.

BONES

Professor Julius Wolff was an orthopaedic surgeon in the 19th century. His work led to Wolff's law which states, 'Bone in a healthy person or animal will adapt to the loads under which it is placed.' What this means is that bones respond positively to stress. Give them more work to do, and they will reinforce and strengthen.

In order for bones to be strengthened, the bone-forming cells called osteoblasts have to be working faster than their colleagues the osteoclasts, which break down bone. Bone breakdown is necessary to release minerals such as calcium which are stored inside. Bones are constantly being broken down and rebuilt, and this process is called 'bone remodelling'.

We reach 90 per cent of our bone mass by the time we're 18. This is why an active childhood is essential. Peak bone mass is reached around the age of 35 and from there it's a slow but steady decline. Around menopause, that bone loss speeds up for a few years. It does then calm down again, but it's still a downward trajectory unless we take action.

> ## GOOD TO KNOW
>
> Oestrogen is crucial when it comes to bone health and is a major player in regulating bone metabolism. There are oestrogen receptors in bone and via these receptors oestrogen can suppress osteoclast activity, which reduces bone breakdown and prolongs the lifespan of the bone-making osteoblast cells. It also helps calcium absorption from the gut, which is a vital mineral for bone creation.

HOW TO STRENGTHEN YOUR BONES

To stimulate the osteoblasts to work harder than the osteoclasts, your bones need to be loaded. Running is an ideal way to do this, because it's a high-impact activity. Every time your foot hits the ground, it sends a jolt or shudder through your bone which triggers the osteoblasts to get to work. Lower-impact activities, such as long walks, swims or bike rides will improve your cardiovascular fitness, but don't seem to provoke an adequate response in bone. You need to hit the ground with more force. Adding rope skipping or jumping drills into your weekly training plan is an excellent way to improve your bone health (see chapter 17).

High-impact activities aren't the only way to stimulate bone growth. Resistance training is really effective, too. Muscles attach to bones via tendons and when you contract a muscle, the tendon tugs on the bone, which stimulates bone formation. As you increase the weight, you get stronger, and a stronger muscle will tug harder on the bone and trigger a greater response. Here are a few things to bear in mind when exercising to increase bone strength:

1. A combination of high-impact, weight-bearing exercise and resistance training works best.
2. Exercise regularly and at least twice per week.
3. You need to challenge your bones to continue strengthening, so keep increasing the workload.
4. Short bursts of activity work well for bone strength, so intervals of exercise followed by rest periods are ideal.

5. Vary the exercise you do. Bones are designed to be strong in a number of directions, so you need to work all your major muscle groups with multi-directional training.
6. Cross training with dancing, tennis or badminton will add to bone strength.
7. Bones can only be made if the building blocks are there. Take a vitamin D tablet daily and make sure your diet is rich in calcium.
8. Bones need adequate recovery to optimise strength.

THE TIPPING POINT

While bones respond well to stress, there is a tipping point where too much challenge causes damage. Injury can also occur if you're missing the other factors needed for good bone health, such as balanced nutrition and good hormonal health or if there are underlying conditions affecting bone strength, such as osteoporosis. The tipping point is different for everyone. There's no generic advice about what duration, frequency and intensity of exercise is too much. Your personal tipping point will change at different times in your life, including in peri- and post-menopause when your bone mass is reducing.

STRESS FRACTURES

Stress fractures develop from overuse. Too much stress on the bone and cracks can form. Common locations for stress fractures in runners include the shins, feet, pelvis and femur (thigh bone).

Running too far, too frequently or increasing your running miles too rapidly can lead to a stress fracture. Recovery is critical, and bones need time to repair and strengthen to adapt to the load you're putting on them. Muscles absorb impact when we run, and weak or fatigued muscles aren't able to absorb as much, which results in extra stress on the bone. You might also be more at risk of a stress fracture if you have poor biomechanics from a muscular imbalance or injury. In this situation, the direction of stress on the bone might not be optimum, leaving it more susceptible to fracture. It's not clear whether different running techniques, such as heel-striking or forefoot running, increase your risk of stress fracture and it's also not clear whether very cushioned shoes will reduce your risk.

How do I know if I've got a stress fracture?

There are warning signs that you might have a stress fracture and if you have any of these you should see your doctor or a physiotherapist. They might need to refer you for x-rays or scans. Stress fractures don't always show up straightaway on an x-ray, so a normal one doesn't always exclude a fracture. Here are the red flags that increase the likelihood of this being a bony injury, rather than a niggle you can run through:

1. Sudden pain – you can pinpoint exactly when the pain started.
2. Worse with activity – the pain doesn't ease up as you run.
3. Pain on resting – it hurts when you're still, particularly pain at night.
4. Point tenderness – you can put your finger on the exact site of the pain.
5. Swelling – injury to bone often causes swelling in the soft tissues around it.
6. Increased risk of bone fracture – you should have a higher index of suspicion if you know you have poor bone health.

Don't run if you think you might have a stress fracture. Use paracetamol and ice packs to relieve pain until you have a diagnosis. Stress fractures take around eight weeks (or more) to heal and you need to rest. You can usually cross train on a static bike if you're pain free, but check with your healthcare professional. Your return to running should be controlled, planned and gradual. It should also only happen once any underlying causes for your stress fracture have been addressed to reduce the risk of it happening again.

OSTEOPOROSIS

Bone density reduces when more is being broken down than being made. Osteopenia is the term used for below-normal bone density, but without correction this can progress to osteoporosis. Bones that are osteoporotic are fragile and break easily. The most commonly affected are the bones in the wrist, hip and spine.

One in two women over 50 experience a bone fracture due to osteoporosis, which can have long-term consequences. If you've never considered osteoporosis before, now is the time to reduce your risk and change your future. A nasty wrist fracture could lead to pain and deformity which affects your career. People who fracture their hip have a 10 to 20 per cent higher risk of dying than expected for their age. When the vertebra in the spine crack and crumble they can compress the spinal nerves, and lead to considerable pain and disability. You can see why this is life-changing stuff.

The most frequently used measure of bone density is a DEXA scan, which compares your bone density to that of a 30-year-old woman. Not everyone needs a DEXA scan, but check if you have any risk factors for osteoporosis (see box below).

When to see your doctor

If any of the following risk factors for osteoporosis apply to you, then it would be a good idea to discuss your bone health. See your doctor if:

- You're over 65.
- Close family members have had osteoporosis.
- Your parent had a hip fracture.
- You smoke.
- You regularly drink more than 14 units of alcohol per week.
- You had your menopause before the age of 45 and aren't using hormone therapy.
- You've used steroid tablets for a medical condition for more than three months in a one-year period.
- You have a bowel condition that affects how nutrients are absorbed by your gut, such as inflammatory bowel disease or coeliac disease.
- You have an overactive thyroid, parathyroid glands or a pituitary gland disorder.

- You're taking a medication that can affect bone strength, such as an anti-oestrogen tablet used after breast cancer.
- You have rheumatoid arthritis.
- You're underweight.
- You have an eating disorder.
- You haven't had a period for more than six months and you aren't pregnant.
- You've had long periods of being inactive, such as bed rest for a long-term condition.
- You've had a bone break after a minor injury.

We can be safe in the knowledge that if we weren't runners, our bone health wouldn't be as good as it is. This is a major reason why it's crucial for us to be able to continue running through menopause. Running less now, when our bones are potentially reducing in density every day, could be detrimental for our future health.

'My GP and I were both shocked when my DEXA scan didn't show any signs of osteoporosis. She'd referred me because in the past I'd had an eating disorder. I've run for 20 years and she suggested that helped improve my bone density. There's no chance I'll ever stop running now!'
Rochelle

Running and osteoporosis

If you've already got a diagnosis of osteoporosis, the good news is that in most cases it's okay to keep running. This is a very individual thing and there are cases, such as with advanced spinal disease or if you've had lots of low-trauma fractures, when the risks of running will outweigh the benefits. Exercise is still really important, though. Speak to your doctor to get advice on what is safe for you. The Royal Osteoporosis Society has a fact sheet on exercising with osteoporosis and a telephone helpline.

Regular running easily covers the recommended guidance of getting 50 impacts with the ground (on each leg) on most days. Resistance exercise will also boost bone formation and balance work will reduce your risk of future falls. Yoga can be very helpful to improve strength and balance, but get advice on which poses are safe for you. Optimise your posture and get advice on how to lift and move correctly. It's safer to avoid exercises that put stress on your spine, such as sit-ups or lifting while bending and twisting. The UK consensus statement on physical activity and exercise for osteoporosis recommends being 'strong, steady and straight' to optimise bone health, reduce risk of falls and improve posture.

Treatments for osteoporosis

If you have osteopenia or osteoporosis, then in addition to increasing your bone strength through exercise, and making sure you have plenty of calcium and vitamin D in your diet, you may be offered medications. HRT is known to strengthen bone and can be used to help prevent osteoporosis developing. Other medications include bisphosphonates, such as alendronic acid or risedronate. Selective oestrogen receptor modulators (SERMs) are another group of medications that help to maintain bone density. In small numbers of people who have severe disease or aren't responding to usual medications, parathyroid hormones or biological medicines might be used. Of course, all these treatments have their specific indications, risks and side-effects, and you need a careful discussion with your doctor about what is right for you.

> 'I have a family history of osteoporosis in my mum and grandmother. I'm on HRT to help prevent loss of bone mass, and I do a lot of weight-bearing and resisted exercise to help too.'
> **Claire Callaghan,** Bristol

JOINTS

Joints are where a bone meets a bone and there are many different types, including ball and socket joints at the hip and shoulder, fixed joints between the skull bones, and hinge joints at the knee, elbow and ankle. Joints are stabilised by ligaments, which run bone to bone, and also by the muscles that surround the joint. Joints are a hive of activity. They're continually being nourished, cleaned up and repaired to keep them working smoothly.

Arthralgia is the medical term for joint pain. If lots of joints are affected it's called polyarthralgia. The knee joint is usually the focus in runners, but hips and ankles are important, too. When perimenopause hits, the issue seems to be more widespread, with many women also complaining of pain in their shoulders, neck and back.

OSTEOARTHRITIS

Osteoarthritis is the most common form of arthritis. It becomes more likely with age and more women are affected than men. The phrase 'wear and tear' arthritis, as it's sometimes called, is unhelpful. It implies we've damaged our joints by being active. I was running on holiday, on a beautiful hot and sunny morning. I ran past a restaurant that was just opening up and one of the staff members shouted out, 'Hey stop running, you'll wreck your knees!' I resisted the temptation to stop and give him a lecture on why this isn't true. This is a very common fear, mostly among those who don't run. Of course, there are caveats, but as recreational, menopausal runners this is not something we need to worry about.

People who are inactive have more problems with their joints than those who are active, including those who run. Osteoarthritis has been found to be less frequent in recreational runners than non-running, sedentary people. The Faculty of Sports and Exercise Medicine statement says, 'Exercise is good for joints and does not cause osteoarthritis.' Importantly, it goes on to say, 'Exercise can help prevent and treat osteoarthritis.' It both reduces pain and improves function.

Runners who already have osteoarthritis in their knees don't have any increased risk of knee pain compared to non-runners and may actually have less. Additionally, studies have shown that runners don't have worse osteoarthritic changes on x-ray compared to non-runners and no worsening if they continue with their running. These study findings are for recreational runners and there may be an increased risk of osteoarthritis for professional and elite athletes.

The main determinant of your osteoarthritis risk is not your running habits, it's your genetics. These dictate how quickly the cartilage, which protects the surface of your bones, wears down. You can't change this. You also can't change the fact you're getting older and you're a woman, both of which increase the risk. There may be a link between declining oestrogen levels in menopause and an increased rate of osteoarthritis developing. Osteoarthritis does, after all, emerge in midlife and more women are affected than men, but more research is needed to fully understand the nature and consequences of any link. Other risk factors for osteoarthritis include being obese, simply because the load on the joints is greater, having a previous joint injury or joint damage from other types of arthritis, such as rheumatoid arthritis.

GOOD TO KNOW

Pain from osteoarthritis tends to get worse as the day goes on and the more you use a joint. It might feel a bit stiff in the morning, but this will only last about half an hour. If you have prolonged morning stiffness and pain, then this is most likely not osteoarthritis. It could be menopause related or, if you have multiple small joints affected with tenderness and swelling, speak to your doctor about the possibility of rheumatoid arthritis, which is an arthritis that needs treatment to prevent it eroding joints.

Please don't stop running in menopause because you're worried about osteoarthritis. Think carefully about what your personal tipping point may be and how you can be as bone friendly as possible. Here are some actions you could take if you think you're at increased risk of osteoarthritis, although they're a pretty sensible action list for all of us, to be honest:

- Reduce the load on your joints by maintaining a healthy weight.
- Move some of your runs onto grass or trail.
- Focus on building muscular strength in your lower legs, so they can absorb more impact.
- Warm up well to ensure muscles are prepped and plenty of synovial fluid is flowing in your joints.
- Set sensible goals and increase your running gradually.
- Include extra rest days to allow bones time to adapt.
- Use clever, low-impact, cross training such as cycling, swimming or rowing to build your cardiovascular fitness.
- Get advice from an expert on your running technique and gait.

When to see your doctor

Working out whether your joint aches and pains are due to menopause or a type of arthritis isn't always easy. See your doctor if:

- You have multiple joints which are giving you pain or stiffness.
- The joints in your hands and feet are affected.
- There's any swelling, tenderness or redness of your joints.
- Morning joint stiffness isn't easing after half an hour.
- Your joint pains restrict your ability to live your daily life.
- Simple painkillers and self-help aren't easing your discomfort.
- You feel unwell with fatigue, fever or loss of appetite.
- You have a family history of rheumatoid arthritis.

SYNOVIAL FLUID

Synovial fluid is very important for joint health in menopause and beyond. Most joints in the body contain synovial fluid, which provides lubrication, but also nourishes the articular cartilage, which covers the bone ends inside the joint. Articular cartilage doesn't have a blood supply, so it's dependent on the synovial fluid to bring it nutrients, and to take away waste products and debris. These processes are regulated by the synovial membrane, which lines the inner surface of the joint capsule. It contains cells, which make synovial fluid and a range of different cells, which work to maintain a healthy joint. Unlike the articular cartilage, the synovial membrane has a blood supply, so it has constant access to nutrients and a way to transport waste away from the joint.

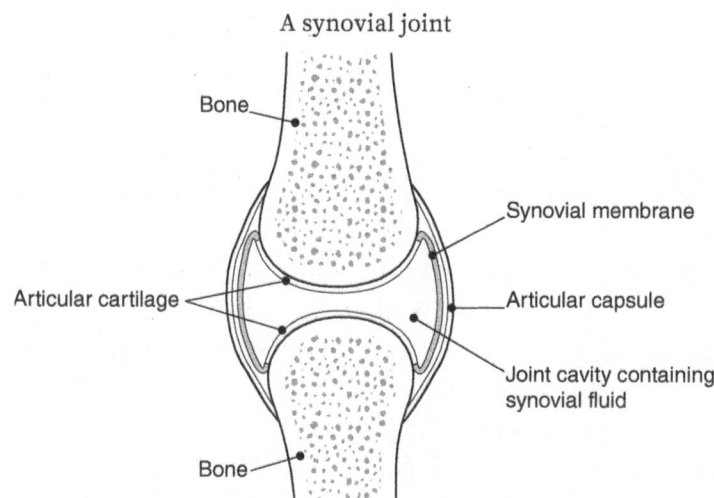

Synovial fluid is largely water, but it contains hyaluronic acid and lubricin for shock absorption and lubrication. It also contains other proteins, enzymes and prostaglandins, which are involved with injury and inflammation in the knee.

Exercise and synovial fluid

A healthy joint needs synovial fluid for joint cartilage to be well nourished, repaired and maintained, and movement to feel comfortable. Exercise stimulates the production of synovial fluid and increases its circulation around the joint. If you're inactive, your joints aren't getting a good wash down with this nutrient-rich fluid. This becomes even more important as we get older, because synovial fluid production slows down, which leads to our joints becoming stiffer and more painful. And to top it all off, it seems that synovial fluid may be altered by the reducing oestrogen levels of menopause too, rather than just by the ageing process. The mechanisms aren't fully understood yet, but oestrogen receptors have been found in synovial tissue, so hormone levels undoubtedly play a role here.

Moving frequently helps to maintain healthy joints. A decent warm-up before the high-impact exercise of running stimulates production and circulation of synovial fluid, which protects our joints. For more about warming up, including a short routine for you to try out, see chapter 17.

LIGAMENTS AND MENOPAUSE

Ligaments attach bone to bone and help to stabilise joints. There are over 900 in the body and they're made of strong connective tissue with lots of collagen fibres. They have a little bit of give in them, but aren't very stretchy. They can be narrow or wide, short or long, depending on their location and function. A sprain happens when a ligament overstretches, such as when you go over on your ankle. Ligaments can also tear or rupture, either partially or fully.

In menopause, lower oestrogen levels result in ligaments becoming stiffer. This may not be a bad thing, because the role of the ligament is to keep a joint stable, stop it dislocating and offer support. A bit less 'give' can be beneficial, and might be one way that our body is adapting and protecting itself against injury as we get older. The story is different when it comes to tendons, but we'll look at those in the next chapter.

GOOD TO KNOW

When you tear a muscle or a tendon it's called a strain. When this happens to a ligament it's called a sprain. There are three grades of sprain. In grade 1, the ligament has been overstretched but there are no tears. Grade 2 sprains have a partial tear in the ligament. In grade 3, the ligament has torn completely, which may mean the joint is unstable.

Plantar fasciitis

Plantar fasciitis (PF) is more common around age 50 in runners and in menopause, so we need to discuss it. While not strictly a ligament, this is a good place to talk about the thick band of fibrous, connective tissue that runs along the sole of your feet, from under your toes to your heel bone. The plantar fascia supports the foot arch and absorbs some of the impact when your foot strikes the ground. When it springs back to its normal shape as your foot leaves the ground, it helps to propel you forwards.

PF, which is inflammation of this band, affects around one in 10 adults, both active and inactive. We don't really understand why it happens. It may be related to tight calf muscles or Achilles tendon thickening. It's definitely linked to increasing running distance too quickly, running biomechanics and possibly the strength of your foot arch. Your shoes can play a role, too – ballet flats have a lot to answer for. The falling oestrogen levels of menopause could be a contributing factor, increasing the likelihood of inflammation, reducing collagen in the tissue and reducing its elasticity. If you gain weight in menopause this can make PF more likely.

PF makes it very painful to put your foot on the ground, although most discomfort is usually around the heel. It's worse when you first get out of bed and when you're barefoot. PF can take six months to a year to resolve. You'll probably have to stop running, at least in the short term, to let the inflammation settle down. Ice packs, anti-inflammatories and heel pads in your shoes can all help ease the pain. Stretching out your calf muscles and the sole of your foot can help, and try rolling a golf ball or frozen water bottle under your foot.

Because the factors that cause PF are so individual, it's ideal to see a physiotherapist to get tailored advice. There are some treatment options, including steroid injections, night splints and shock wave therapy, but results can be varied.

HOW TO SOOTHE YOUR ACHING JOINTS

It's difficult to keep moving when everything really hurts. Think about what you can do rather than what you can't. Any movement is good, however gentle. Ease your pain a bit before you move with a warm bath or painkiller. Start with walking to get the synovial fluid circulating, then do some gentle mobility exercises. Even if it causes a bit of pain or discomfort it will still be beneficial for your joints. Hopefully you'll feel more comfortable after this. That might be enough for you and it's fine to leave it there. Use your better days to do a bit more and try a run when you feel able, but don't be tempted to overdo it. You need to find the right balance between activity and rest, and this can be a tricky, moving target in menopause, so it's important to be flexible with your routines.

Hormone therapy can reduce the symptoms of musculoskeletal syndrome of menopause, and many women say that it enables them to be active, because of the effect it has on their joints.

I'm not pretending that what you eat will rid you of all your pain, but there's lots you can do with your nutrition to help look after your bones and joints. Including lots of anti-inflammatory foods and omega-3 fatty acids, such as those in fish oils, flax and chia seeds, is a great place to start. Take your daily vitamin D and consider using bovine collagen supplements (see chapter 16). There's no overwhelming evidence that other supplements, including glucosamine, chondroitin and curcumin, which is the active ingredient in turmeric, will help. Some women report they do, so assuming they're safe for you, there's usually no harm in trying. For more about using supplements safely, see chapter 16.

CHAPTER 11

Muscles and Tendons

There's a reason why your social media feeds are full of Lycra-clad influencers flinging weights around. Over recent years it's become really clear that muscles do much more than move our body around. They're an important key to good present and future health. Muscles can, however, cause a few issues in menopause, which directly affect our running. Having a good understanding of our muscles will help us to overcome these barriers and stay motivated to keep working them hard, even if we don't really enjoy strength work! If we don't take action and look after our muscles, it will almost certainly have a negative impact on our health.

MUSCLES FOR HEALTH

When you exercise a muscle, it releases proteins called myokines. Some myokines stay in muscle tissue and others move into the bloodstream. There are hundreds of types of myokine and they have different functions in the body, including acting as anti-inflammatories. Even a short run causes myokine release and they'll stay in your circulation for an hour or so afterwards. In some studies, myokine levels didn't return to baseline until 24 hours after exercise. Most of the major chronic diseases, such as heart disease, type 2 diabetes and cancer, are partly due to a low level of inflammation in the body. This is called chronic systemic inflammation. Exercising regularly ensures there are plenty of anti-inflammatory myokines in our circulation, which will reduce our risk of major diseases. When we're inactive, fewer myokines are released and the body seems to become more resistant to them, too. This results in inflammation levels rising, which leads to muscle breakdown, increased visceral fat levels and increased insulin resistance. The result is a higher risk of disease, particularly type 2 diabetes.

Age is our biggest risk factor for these major diseases and most people become less active as they age. Muscles can directly reduce the chances of us being diagnosed with many medical conditions. That's powerful stuff! Rather than less, we really need to do more exercise as we move through into post-menopause. There's research underway to work out which types of exercise release which types of myokines and what the effect of those is on our health. I think it's super-interesting!

Muscles for independence

Muscles keep us mobile and balanced, which is important for running. We've all tripped on a paving slab, stumbled on a tree root or slipped in some mud. We can usually keep our balance and run on without injury, but without strong muscles the story can be very different.

The NHS says that one in three adults over 65 and half of those over 80 will have at least one fall a year. Falls can be catastrophic for health, leading to head injuries, hip fractures and the inability to live independently. Around a third of people who have a hip fracture die within 12 months and 10 to 20 per cent of people who have previously lived at home require nursing-home care after a hip fracture. I make no apologies for giving you these stark facts. We need to know this. If nothing else it can act as motivation to exercise.

Recent data shows a sharp increase in the rate of falls in women after age 40. We need to take action now to reduce our risk of falls in the future. This isn't something that just affects old people. Regular exercise can reduce the risk of falls by around one-third. Good balance is important, but so is muscle strength. From the small muscles in our feet and ankles to our major postural muscles, we need them all. Our ability to remain steady on a forward lunge could be the thing that stops us toppling over and fracturing our hip when we stumble age 80.

Muscles for metabolism

Muscles have an influence on our body's metabolism (see chapter 12). Many women complain of increasing levels of body fat during perimenopause and muscle mass is part of the cause and solution to this. Muscles are also a fuel source, taking up glucose after we've eaten and storing it as glycogen, so it's available for our body to use in between meals and when we exercise. If we're fasted and glycogen stores are depleted, then the body turns to other stores including muscle protein.

Sarcopenia

It's clear that after our mid-thirties, when age-related muscle loss begins, the state of our muscles can determine our general health, and some studies show a slight acceleration in muscle loss around menopause. Sarcopenia is the term used for this condition of low muscle mass related to ageing, with losses of up to 1 per cent per year. It has its biggest impact when we're old, leading to frailty, disability and an increased risk of chronic disease.

Let's dive a bit deeper into muscle loss. There are different types of muscle, but the one we're talking about here is skeletal muscle, which is made up of bundles of muscle fibres. There are several types of muscle fibre, including type 1, also called slow-twitch muscle fibres, which give us endurance, and type 2, which are fast-twitch fibres, giving us speed and power for sprints and jumps. As we lose muscle mass, the fibres decline in both size and number. More of the fast-twitch fibres are lost than the slow-twitch, which explains why we notice our running speed declining. Fat cells begin to infiltrate the muscle tissue and the number of satellite cells, which help to repair and regenerate muscle fibres after we've worked out, reduce in number.

Although sarcopenia is an involuntary loss, there are causative factors that we can influence. We can slow or even reverse muscle loss. Here are some of the reasons that sarcopenia develops:

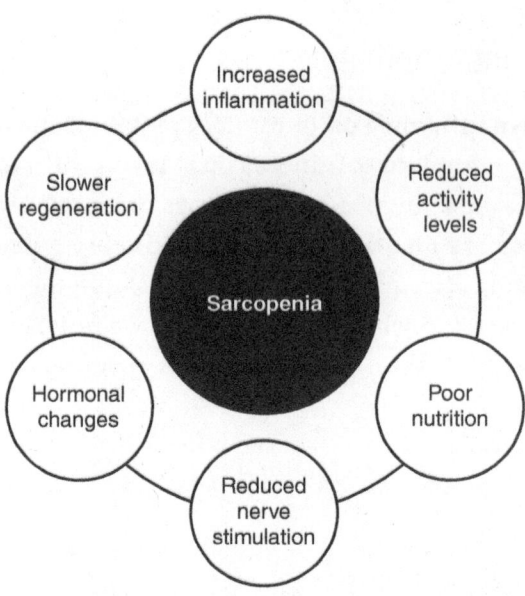

- Reduced activity levels – people commonly move less with age.
- Poor nutrition – insufficient calories, particularly inadequate protein intake, but also obesity where high numbers of fat cells within muscles can accelerate muscle loss.
- Reduced nerve stimulation – fewer neuromuscular junctions where nerves connect with muscles and stimulate them to contract, especially in fast-twitch fibres.
- Hormonal change – reducing levels of insulin-like growth factor, oestrogen and testosterone probably all influence sarcopenia.
- Increased inflammation – more chronic systemic inflammation in our bodies as we get older, particularly if we have any medical conditions. Lower oestrogen levels might contribute to this, too.
- Slower regeneration – older muscle can't repair and regenerate as quickly for many reasons, including reduced function and number of the mitochondria, which supply energy to muscle cells, and a reduced lifespan of muscle cells.

Addressing these factors will help you prevent sarcopenia. Maintaining or increasing your activity levels and improving your nutrition, particularly making sure you eat enough protein, is key. Looking after yourself generally to reduce your risk of chronic diseases is important, too. Using our muscles triggers release of anti-inflammatory proteins, so it becomes an upwards spiral if we take action and a downwards spiral if we don't. There isn't enough evidence yet to prescribe HRT purely for sarcopenia prevention, but there may be drugs developed in the future to target those more molecular changes that affect muscle regeneration. We're living longer and that can mean more sarcopenia and frailty, so this is an important area of research, but it's clear that we need to maintain the muscle we already have and build more to set us up for a healthy future (see chapter 19).

> 'I go to a weight training class once or twice a week to strengthen my muscles, along with a pilates class. I also regularly cycle and walk, as well as run.'
> **Hilary**

Common Muscle Problems

Myalgia

Myalgia is the medical term for aching and painful muscles. It's common in menopause and is a big part of the musculoskeletal syndrome of menopause. You may find that you're achier than you used to be, get muscle soreness more quickly and that your muscles take longer to recover. It's one of those symptoms that can make you feel 'old'.

Heat, massage or simple painkillers ease muscle pains, and swimming, some gentle yoga or a walk can give relief to low-level pain. Some women find HRT helps and allows them to be more active, which in turn helps to loosen their muscles. Managing training can be difficult, and requires patience and flexibility. You may need to add extra rest days or increase your training more slowly. Turn to chapter 17 to read more about adapting your training in menopause.

GOOD TO KNOW

When you have a musculoskeletal injury, taking a non-steroidal anti-inflammatory drug (NSAID) such as ibuprofen can quickly help to ease pain and reduce inflammation, but it may not be the best thing to use. In this setting, inflammation is helpful, it brings healing cells to the damaged tissues and activates satellite cells which regenerate muscle. If you delay or dampen that process with an NSAID, then repair will be slower and possibly less effective. NSAIDs can also affect collagen production and impair repair of damaged tendons and ligaments, too. If you need to take pain relief for an injury, paracetamol is felt to be a better choice.

Fibromyalgia

Fibromyalgia is a condition that affects around one in 20 people in the UK. The symptoms are very similar to the perimenopause and they usually start in midlife. Here are some of the common symptoms:

- Stiff and painful muscles, which can ache, burn or throb.
- Extreme fatigue.
- Disturbed sleep.
- Brain fog.
- Headaches.
- Numbness or tingling in arms or legs.
- Restless legs.
- Increased sensitivity to touch, light, noise, smells or heat.
- Digestive problems such as abdominal pain, bloating and constipation.
- Painful periods.
- Low mood, usually as a result of other symptoms.

It's easy to confuse fibromyalgia and menopause, especially as they may both happen at the same time. Symptoms can get worse with the weather, with stress and just out of the blue. The cause of fibromyalgia is unknown, but it does tend to run in families. The risk of having it increases if you have certain other medical conditions, such as rheumatoid or osteoarthritis, lupus or irritable bowel syndrome. In some people, symptoms begin after an emotional or physical trigger, such as an accident, operation or infection. It's thought that it may originate from the brain and nervous system with changes in the messages between nerve cells that process pain. Fibromyalgia is 'a diagnosis of exclusion', which means having tests and investigations to rule out other causes before the diagnosis can be made.

Fibromyalgia is difficult to treat. There's a focus on helping you to remain active, which is hard if you're in pain. It also centres on a psychological approach using talking therapies and antidepressants to help improve quality of life by reducing pain, helping sleep and supporting mental health.

There are women who are given a diagnosis of fibromyalgia without considering that their symptoms may be due to menopause and, conversely, some women are told their symptoms are 'just menopause' when in fact it's fibromyalgia. It's important to consider both, because the diagnosis directs the treatment. There are so many unknowns in this area of medicine, so share your learnings and concerns with your doctor.

GOOD TO KNOW

It's reported that throughout life, women experience more pain than men and many more women than men are being treated for long-term pain conditions. Hormone fluctuations are thought to affect the way we perceive and experience pain, both during our menstrual cycle and in menopause. Oestrogen levels can influence the release of and response to endorphins, the body's natural painkillers. Women who have lots of menopause symptoms have been found to have a higher risk of chronic pain. Other factors affect how much pain we feel in menopause, with sleep deprivation and high stress levels known to lower the threshold at which we feel pain.

> 'I've always strength-trained in some form, so I haven't noticed a deterioration in muscle mass. If anything, it's increased over the past nine months due to sticking to a set programme and routine. I'd fully recommend strength training alongside running to lessen the chance of injury, maintain or increase performance, or just to feel a little bit awesome!'
> **Sarah**

Muscle cramps

Lots of women get muscle cramps once they hit perimenopause. They can affect sleep if they're happening at night, perhaps as part of restless legs syndrome (see chapter 4). This impairs running recovery and performance, and a strong muscle cramp in your leg can still feel sore and painful to run on the next day. Some women find they cramp up more easily during running, which can be frustrating.

During a cramp, the muscle fibres get stuck in a contracted state and can't relax. We don't really understand why muscle cramps increase during menopause. We know there are oestrogen receptors in muscles and tendons, and musculoskeletal tissues are changing generally during menopause. There may be lifestyle triggers, so look at your daily life and exercise schedule to see if anything has changed. Are you more or less active than you used to be? Are you really well hydrated and well nourished before, during and after exercise? Dehydration and electrolyte imbalance can cause muscle cramps, especially on long runs on hot days. Do you have other symptoms that might suggest the cramps are part of something wider, such as iron deficiency, a thyroid disorder or a trapped nerve? If so, see your doctor for an assessment.

When you get a muscle cramp, alongside swearing loudly, try and passively stretch the affected muscle. For a calf cramp, take hold of your foot or put a scarf around the ball of your foot and draw it towards you. I get random toe cramps and holding the toe and gently moving it helps. You might need to get up, walk around and breathe deeply. You can try gently massaging a cramped muscle or applying hot or cold compresses, but they usually settle on their own.

Low back pain

More women than men get low back pain. The risk increases with age, but the group most likely to be affected at any one time is people aged 41 to 50. In women, it's hard to know how much of this is directly due to menopause, and how much is due to age and lifestyle factors. There have been studies which show that women who have premature menopause are more likely to get low back pain, but the exact reason for this is not known. There has also been research that shows women who have higher levels of psychological stress during midlife have more back pain. It's most likely a multitude of factors, including the changing musculoskeletal system in menopause, altered lifestyle habits and hormonal influences on pain perception.

Active recovery rather than excessive rest is encouraged for back pain now. Simple low back pain usually settles in a few weeks, and you should try to keep active and continue your daily routine as much as possible. Running is not advised. Wait until you feel comfortable walking. Paracetamol isn't routinely recommended for low back pain anymore. Instead use heat packs and back exercises, and if you need pain relief, then use ibuprofen if it's safe for you to take.

The key for back pain is prevention. That means strengthening your back muscles, and learning to move and lift in a way that protects your back. You can access exercises via a group programme or consider seeing a physiotherapist for individual advice. Pilates is a very effective way to build up your core strength and protect your back. You'll need to continue doing back exercises on a regular basis to minimise the risk of back pain returning.

> 'I have a spondylolisthesis and used to get back pain with running. A strengthening regime and physiotherapy has addressed this, and now my back pain is almost non-existent.'
> **Claire Callaghan,** Bristol

When to see your doctor

Most back pain settles in a few weeks with self-care, but there are some red flags that might indicate more serious causes of back pain, including cauda equina syndrome, which can cause permanent nerve damage. See your doctor if:

- Your pain is no better after three to four weeks or it has become more severe in the meantime.
- You have pain radiating down both legs.
- You have any weakness of your legs and can't move them normally.
- You aren't able to pass urine or have been incontinent of urine or faeces.
- You feel numb and have lost sensation around your anus or in the perineum (area between your vagina and anus).
- You feel unwell generally or have a high temperature.
- You're losing weight unexpectedly.
- You have other medical issues, such as diabetes or a previous history of cancer.

Piriformis syndrome

Another muscle-related issue that's common in women over 50 and in runners too is piriformis syndrome. The piriformis muscle sits behind your gluteus maximus muscle and runs from your lower spine to the top of your thigh bone. It helps to turn your leg outwards and rotate your hip. If it becomes tight or goes into spasm it can cause buttock pain. It can also squash the sciatic nerve, which runs close by, and causes pain, tingling and numbness down the back of your leg. The pain from piriformis syndrome can be triggered by prolonged sitting, running up hill and going downstairs. Treatment focuses on identifying and reducing triggers, stretching the piriformis muscle and strengthening the hip muscles.

Tendons

Tendons are bands of thick, collagen-rich connective tissue that attach muscles to bones. This is handy when there are lots of bulky muscles and not much space, such as in the shoulder joint. When you contract a muscle, the tendon transfers the energy the muscle is generating to the bone. Tendons give a little, but they aren't stretchy. Less energy would be transferred if they were. They don't tear easily, but they can get strained and when they're injured they can take a long time to heal, partly because they don't have a very rich blood supply.

Like ligaments, tendons become stiffer in menopause. While this can be helpful for joint-stabilising ligaments, it's not such good news for tendons. A stiffer tendon 'gives' less and the risk of injury is higher in post-menopausal women than it is in pre-menopause. Tendons which are particularly vulnerable are those in the hips and shoulders, and the Achilles tendon. The gluteal and hamstring tendons are often affected, too.

Tendon repair can take longer after menopause, with lower oestrogen levels resulting in a slower turnover of collagen fibres and reduced tendon strength. This is another reason we need to ensure we increase our training gradually and include enough rest days to allow for tendon recovery. It also means that recovery after an injury may take longer than it has done previously for us or compared to men.

Obesity is a significant risk factor for tendon problems due to an increased load on tendons and possibly due to higher inflammation levels caused by obesity, too.

Whether tendon problems can be reduced by using HRT is a largely unanswered question. A study of post-menopausal women with tendon-related hip pain done in 2021 did show some improvement after 12 weeks in women with a low to normal body mass index (BMI) who were using hormone therapy alongside exercise and education. The study was small and did have limitations, but it indicates there may be some benefits to using HRT in tendon-related hip pain. More studies are needed to confirm this and to look at other tendons too.

Common tendon-related problems

With oestrogen levels influencing the health of our tendons, and tendon issues being more frequent in runners, it's easy to see why tendon-related problems are common in menopausal runners. To run and strength train effectively, efficiently and safely, you need full use of your upper and lower body, so a tendon issue anywhere can be problematic. To treat tendon injuries and return to running as soon as possible, it's advisable to see a physiotherapist to confirm the diagnosis and give you graded exercises to support tendon healing and strengthening.

Listed here are some common tendon-related issues that affect women during the menopause transition and have a significant knock-on effect to training.

Frozen shoulder

A frozen shoulder is most common in women between 40 and 60, and more likely in people who have diabetes or have had a shoulder injury. Also called adhesive capsulitis, frozen shoulder is a condition that causes pain, stiffness and reduced shoulder movement. It begins with inflammation followed by thickening and constriction of the soft tissues of the shoulder. There are three phases:

- Freezing – pain is the main symptom.
- Frozen – stiffness is prominent but pain has reduced.
- Thawing – things gradually return to normal.

Pain relief and physiotherapy will help the shoulder be as mobile as possible, and steroid injections can be effective. It can take many months or even years to go away, but it usually does, eventually. You can continue to run with a frozen shoulder, but be aware that your arm swing may be affected by limited shoulder movements.

> 'Experiencing a frozen shoulder during perimenopause was painful and restrictive, significantly affecting my running and daily life. After a small procedure and starting HRT, it's settled down and I'm back to running comfortably. I've learned this symptom is common, yet many women don't realise it's linked to menopause.'
> **Mel Bound**

Achilles tendinopathy

The Achilles is the strongest and longest tendon in the body. It connects your calf muscles to your heel bone. Achilles tendinopathy doesn't seem to be directly linked to menopause and is more common in men. It does, however, affect people between ages 30 and 50 and is more common in runners than non-runners. New runners or those suddenly increasing their running miles, especially with lots of fast running or hilly terrain, are most at risk.

In Achilles tendinopathy the Achilles tendon becomes painful, stiff and weak in response to overload or repetitive strain. It may be swollen and tender to touch. Pain and stiffness is usually worse in the morning, if you've been still for a while and before or straight after a run.

Reducing and spacing your activity is usually preferable to stopping. Avoid wearing flat and unsupportive footwear – a heel-lift shoe insert can help. Specific stretching and strengthening exercises, including 'eccentric' exercises (where you're loading a muscle as it lengthens), are very important. It may clear in a few weeks, but can take up to six months or longer, and sometimes surgery is required, but it shouldn't be ignored as it can progress to tendon rupture.

Gluteal tendinopathy

This tendon attaches your gluteal muscles to the top of your thigh bone. It's a common cause of pain on the outside of the hip and is more common during menopause. Around one in four women over the age of

50 have experienced this, but there are lots of causes of hip pain, so it's important to get a diagnosis from a medical professional.

If it is inflamed or injured, the gluteal tendon can become painful. This can be due to overuse, so it's common in runners. It can be caused by underuse, too. Pain tends to focus on the upper, outer part of your thigh bone and can extend down the outside of your leg. Sometimes you can feel it in your low back, groin or in the glutes themselves. Sitting with your legs crossed or lying on your side in bed at night causes pain.

Treatment focuses on exercises which strengthen the glutes, hip muscles and tendons. Pace and space your activity, increase what you're doing gradually and allow enough recovery days. Avoiding triggers that cause pain, such as sitting cross-legged, or avoiding lots of hills or stairs can help.

Complete rest is not advised. Try cross training rather than running while you are in pain to reduce the load on the hips. Most cases will have settled within one year, but with treatment it can be quicker than that.

Proximal hamstring tendinopathy (PHT)

The hamstrings are the muscles at the back of the thigh. They run from the ischial tuberosity (your sitting bone) down to the lower leg. This type of tendinopathy is common in runners and women, and it increases with age, so it's important for us to know about.

PHT affects the hamstring tendons at the ischial tuberosity. They are thick, fibrous and have a poor blood supply. Multiple factors contribute to PHT including excessive training, being overweight, and weak leg, hip and core muscles. Pain is usually felt deep in the buttock and back of the thigh. It's worse after running, squatting and sitting. An MRI scan is often needed to differentiate PHT from other causes of buttock and leg pain.

Avoid activities that exacerbate pain or cause pain for several days after doing them. Running on the flat might feel alright, but cross train if running is making your pain worse. Exercises from a physiotherapist will help to reduce pain, and strengthen the muscles and tendons, but don't be tempted to keep stretching your hamstrings in the early days as it can make things worse. There's no quick fix, but you should hope to be back to normal in three to six months. Take care with hill running and speed sessions, though, as these are most likely to aggravate PHT.

Carpal tunnel syndrome

Carpal tunnel syndrome is a nerve condition rather than a tendon one, but it can be caused by swollen tendons and I want to include it because it's very common in women (three times more than in men), particularly in peri- and post-menopause.

The median nerve becomes squashed as it travels through a tunnel in the wrist, which can easily become narrowed by swelling of the surrounding structures, including the wrist tendons. Excessive or repetitive wrist movement can cause tendon swelling. It's common in pregnancy, diabetes and thyroid disorders, and can be hereditary, too. Pain, numbness and tingling is felt in the hand, usually the thumb, index, middle and ring fingers, and pain may radiate up the forearm. It comes on gradually and can be very severe, usually getting worse at night and badly affecting sleep.

It's important to get treated to avoid permanent damage to the nerve and the muscles it supplies. A wrist splint and avoiding activities that exacerbate it can ease pain. Simple painkillers can help and sometimes a steroid injection into the wrist is needed. Surgery to relieve the pressure on the nerve by releasing the top of the carpal tunnel is frequently done when symptoms aren't settling.

Night pain will resolve within a few days of surgery, but numbness and recovering strength in the wasted hand muscles can take many months. Take a couple of weeks off running after surgery to allow stitches to heal. After that, it's really determined by pain levels and your confidence, which can be low if you're worried about tripping and falling on your wrist.

CHAPTER 12

Body Composition

One of the biggest complaints I hear from women in menopause is that their body shape is changing and they don't like it. Despite running and eating as normal, their clothes stop fitting and they don't recognise the silhouette in the mirror. This can happen gradually or suddenly and unexpectedly. It can lower self-esteem and confidence, and add to the feeling of loss of control. It's easy to become frustrated with your body, especially if the steps you take to regain control don't work. These body changes impact our running and our health.

Most women gain a bit of weight with age and it's not all down to hormones. The Study of Women's Health Across the Nation (SWAN) is research based in the United States, and it's looking at the health and quality of life of a large group of women from diverse backgrounds as they move through midlife. They've found that midlife is a time when women gain weight, but this starts before menopause hormone changes begin. Their data showed weight goes up gradually at a rate of 0.7 kilograms per year and doesn't spike during perimenopause.

If weight gain in midlife is mostly due to ageing, then why does your body start changing shape when you hit perimenopause? SWAN found that during perimenopause and for about two years after the last menstrual period, body composition changes accelerate. Body composition is the relative amounts of fat, muscle, bone and water that make up your body. This large study found that during the menopause transition, women gained body fat and lost lean muscle mass. The rate of fat gain doubled from that of pre-menopause, with total body-fat mass increasing around 2 per cent per year. Any weight gain from increased fat was balanced by the amount of muscle lost.

There are differences between racial groups, though. The patterns of weight gain and body composition changes were similar in black and white women, while Japanese women lost muscle mass but didn't gain fat mass during menopause and Chinese women seemed to lose fat mass, gain muscle and lose weight in the post-menopause phase. Interestingly, having a later menopause seemed to make body composition changes and weight gain less severe.

> ## GOOD TO KNOW
>
> When does it all end? From about two years after your last menstrual period, body composition changes start to stabilise. Weight gain slows and stops. It's important to remember this doesn't go on forever, though, because this is a transition phase and we move into a new steady state in post-menopause.

This conversation is very much about body composition and not about weight. Whatever weight, size or shape you are at the start of perimenopause, this is your opportunity to think about health over weight. A static number on the scales may be falsely reassuring and not reflect what's going on inside you. Your body composition is changing, and this can have negative health consequences, so action is needed. If you're focusing solely on trying to reduce the number on the scales, you can end up feeling like a failure when this doesn't budge. Using weight loss as a marker of your health can be very misleading. Your weight may go up, yet your body composition may improve with an increased muscle mass and lower fat stores. Similarly, your weight may go down, but that doesn't necessarily mean you're healthier. If you're overweight or obese, there are well-known health benefits from losing weight, but when it comes to menopause it's vital to understand that making positive lifestyle changes such as exercising regularly will improve your health regardless of what the scales say. If you're doing the work, you will be healthier on the inside.

Alongside the increased body-fat percentage during menopause is a change in where fat gets laid down. More fat gets deposited around the middle of the body. Previously fat might have settled around your hips and thighs, giving what's classified as a 'pear shape'. In menopause, however, with more fat being laid down around your waist, your body can become more of an 'apple shape'. I don't like being compared to a piece of fruit to be honest, but it helps to picture the change. Women say their waist feels thick and solid. It's not just squishy fat under the skin, but a firmness and fullness indicating deeper fat deposition.

> 'I look at myself in the mirror and wonder who the hell is this woman?! The belly fat irks me the most. I've always had a tiny waist and thunder thighs, now it looks like my belly is catching up with them. And you'd think my boobs would plump up with this, but nope, those look baggy and saggy, too.'
> **Carri Ables**

WHY DOES IT HAPPEN?

There are some clear reasons related to ageing and lifestyle which drive weight and body composition changes, and there are numerous theories relating to hormonal influences. It's likely to be a combination of all of them and also of processes that haven't been discovered yet. Here are some of the factors at play:

- **Activity levels**: Chances are, aside from your running, you're now less active day to day and spend more time sitting than you did 10 years ago, although, of course, this depends on your job and family life. Senior work roles are often more desk-based and you're probably no longer running around after children all day. If you're more tired in the evenings, you might spend longer watching TV. These changes can be so gradual and subtle that you don't realise they're happening. Even a small change in activity level over a long period of time makes a difference to how much fat our body stores. When we sit for more than around 20 minutes, our metabolism switches into storage mode. Enzymes such as lipoprotein lipase, which break down fat, switch off. The biggest increase is in the amount of visceral fat, a harmful fat which I'll explain in a moment.

- **Basal metabolic rate (BMR)**: Our BMR is the energy our body uses to keep ticking over and includes the energy needed for breathing, heart function and digestion. As we get older, our BMR reduces. This is largely due to a decline in muscle mass; muscles use a lot of energy so with less of them, our body doesn't require as much. With a lower baseline energy requirement from the body, even when we're resting, it's easy to end up with excess energy (calories) which gets stored as fat.
- **Hormonal changes**: When ovarian function declines, the production of oestrodiol reduces and the main source of oestrogen switches to oestrone from the adrenals and fat cells (see chapter 1). One theory is that the body intentionally lays down more fat cells to produce oestrone and top up body oestrogen levels. FSH rises sharply to stimulate oestrogen production when perimenopause begins. Increased central body-fat changes begin before oestrogen levels have really declined, suggesting that FSH might be more important than previously thought.
- **Appetite changes**: Oestrogen influences the release and effect of hunger hormones. It suppresses ghrelin, the hunger-stimulating hormone and lower levels of oestrogen result in higher levels of ghrelin, meaning you're hungrier and potentially eating more. It may also be the ratio and balance of oestrogen with progesterone and testosterone, both of which can stimulate appetite. It's confusing and we don't have all the answers, but an increase in appetite is common in menopause and can lead to increased body-fat levels.
- **Stress levels**: Cortisol is our stress hormone. Short bursts of it are helpful, ensuring we can be alert and function at our best under pressure. Continuously high cortisol levels from longer-term stress encourage our body to store energy as fat, in preparation for more stressful times ahead. In addition to work, family and

relationship stress, exercise can cause stress, too. It's not the brief bursts of cortisol from a high-intensity workout that we need to worry about, they're fine and shouldn't be avoided, it's our overall training schedule and the balance between activity, energy and recovery. Insufficient rest and not supplying our body with the energy it needs for our exercise will stress it, raise cortisol and potentially increase body fat. This is why training harder, longer or fasted might not result in the reduction of weight or body fat that we expect. Exercise can be hard to fit in and can itself feel like an added pressure. If we end up exercising less, we'll probably gain weight and body fat. Lots of women turn to food as a comfort at times of stress or have less time and energy to eat well. It's easy to see why stress can be a big player in a changing body shape.

- **Sleep:** Being awake for longer and moving more as a result, may mean you use up more calories daily. If worry and anxiety keep you awake, the mental energy required for that can also result in weight loss. However, long-term lack of sleep causes stress, raises cortisol levels and increases body fat. Sleep deprivation increases ghrelin levels, which stimulates appetite and it suppresses leptin levels, so you don't feel full. It can also affect insulin sensitivity, increasing the risk of developing type 2 diabetes. Data from the Nurses' Health Study found that, over the course of the 16-year study, women who slept less than six hours per night gained 1.1 kilograms (2.5 pounds) more than those who slept for seven hours per night. Confusingly, people who sleep for more than 10 hours per night are more likely to be obese.

> 'My body has changed very little over the decades, apart from a few more wrinkles. I wonder if this is because I've trained hard and eaten well consistently throughout my life?'
> **Sarah Jones,** Isle of Wight

WHAT ARE THE CONSEQUENCES?

Do these body composition changes matter? Their impact is not insignificant, and they can affect our physical and mental health. The consequences of a falling muscle mass include an increased risk of multiple medical conditions, a lower chance of living independently in old age and detrimental effects on our running (see chapter 11). A rising body-fat percentage and a higher bodyweight also increase our risk of long-term medical conditions and make running harder, because more effort is required. Additionally, we might feel self-conscious about the way we look. Let's not pretend that it's easy for all of us to be proud of our new shape. It's a complicated and very personal issue, and we all approach it differently. Ultimately, though, if we're running and exercising less as a result of changes to our body shape, this has a huge impact on all areas of our health. Taking action is not just about aesthetics, it's about addressing our present and future health.

Body fat

Our body-fat levels are determined by our genetics, age, ethnicity, diet and physical activity levels. Women generally have a higher body-fat percentage than men. What constitutes a healthy body varies between individuals. For women it's said to be between 15 and 31 per cent, but it may be a little higher for women over 40. For men, it's between 18 and 25 per cent.

There are two main types of body fat: subcutaneous fat, which is stored just under the skin, and visceral fat which is stored in and around internal organs such as the heart, liver and muscles. Subcutaneous fat keeps us warm, protects our bones and cushions us from impact. Fat is a wonderful energy supplier, and it can store and release energy as and when we need it, which is crucial to us as runners.

Visceral fat

Visceral fat is metabolically very active, which means it releases hormones and other chemicals which influence processes in the body. It also causes inflammation, which we know contributes to disease. High levels of visceral fat put us at greater risk of a number of health conditions, including:

- Metabolic syndrome.
- Type 2 diabetes.
- Increased insulin resistance.
- Cardiovascular disease, including heart attacks and strokes.
- Certain cancers, including breast and bowel cancer.

You can't tell how much visceral fat someone has by looking at them. Someone with a larger waist probably has more visceral fat than someone with a smaller one, but it's not always the case. A woman with low levels of subcutaneous fat can still have high levels of visceral fat. It's crucial not to make judgements about someone's health by simply looking at their size.

> ### GOOD TO KNOW
> Weighing scales that measure body composition, including fancy ones at the gym, aren't very accurate. They're also poor at differentiating between visceral and subcutaneous fat. These smart scales can, however, be useful to give you a baseline if you're wanting to change your body composition. You can take serial measurements and look for trends. Some 3D scans available in the community can be valid, but the most accurate results of body composition come from medical scans, including MRI and DEXA scans.

'A belly and thick waist appeared out of nowhere in about three months! I now only wear leggings with a wide high waistband to stop it all rolling over the top and digging in. Yuck!'

Anonymous

Oestrogen levels influence what type of fat is stored where in the body. As oestrogen levels fall, fat is more likely to be deposited around the middle of the body and visceral fat levels increase from around 5 to 8 per cent of bodyweight to around 10 to 15 per cent from pre- to post-menopause. FSH may have an influence here and more research is needed to determine exactly how the sex hormones affect fat deposition.

A quick word about adiponectin. This is a hormone made and secreted by fat cells. It's just one of many adipocytokines, which are the messengers sent out from fat cells, which influence our metabolism. Adiponectin is still being researched, but it appears to have various roles, including increasing the body's sensitivity to insulin. This is important because insulin controls our blood glucose (sugar) levels. If insulin sensitivity falls and the body becomes resistant to insulin, type 2 diabetes develops. Adiponectin encourages fat to be stored as the healthier subcutaneous fat rather than as visceral fat. It also helps to suppress inflammation in the body, which reduces the risk of many medical conditions. Adiponectin levels are lower in people with type 2 diabetes, obesity and cardiovascular disease.

There's still a lot we don't know about adiponectin. Some studies have shown that adiponectin levels fall during perimenopause and gradually increase again in post-menopause. This is likely to be linked to our changing hormonal status, but the exact mechanism isn't fully understood. At a basic level it would seem to make sense that some of the changes we see in our bodies during menopause, such as increased visceral fat and increased insulin resistance, are linked to lower adiponectin levels. So how do we increase them? The answers aren't clear yet, but regular exercise and eating a healthy, balanced diet, such as the Mediterranean diet, are currently our best bet.

Visceral fat is generally very responsive to exercise and, alongside a decent diet, moving more is a great way to reduce it. Again, regardless of what the scales say, if you're exercising regularly you will be getting healthier from the inside out.

Remember that low body-fat levels can be harmful, too. Fat isn't all bad and it's needed for normal bodily function. Low body-fat levels can lead to issues which affect women in pre-menopause such as amenorrhoea (absent periods) with an effect on fertility, but it's still important in post-menopause with persistent low body-fat levels putting you at risk of developing osteoporosis, nutritional deficiencies and an impaired immune system.

> ## GOOD TO KNOW
>
> If you're trying to assess or reduce your central body fat, weighing scales probably aren't your best indicator. Body mass index (BMI) which looks at your weight relative to your height is also unhelpful, because it doesn't take body composition into account. Aside from 3D scans, your best tool is a tape measure.
>
> Waist-to-height or waist-to-hip ratios are simple and useful measurements for assessing how much fat you have around the middle of your body and, in turn, your risk of health conditions such as type 2 diabetes and cardiovascular disease. There are situations where these are less accurate, such as if you have a very high BMI.
>
> - **Waist-to-height ratio:** Measure the narrowest part of your waist and divide it by your height. A waist-to-height ratio of greater than 0.5 is a sign that you have more central fat and an increased risk. Basically, your waist should be less than half your height.
> - **Waist-to-hip ratio:** Measure the narrowest part of your waist and divide it by the widest part of your hips and bum. A waist-to-hip ratio of greater than 0.85 in women is a sign that you have more central fat and an increased risk.

HOW MUCH DO YOU SIT?

Increased sedentary time is an important reason why body composition changes happen and the risk of type 2 diabetes increases. This is still relevant to you if you have an active job. When we sit for longer than about half an hour, our metabolism changes. It switches from active and using energy to inactive and storing energy. This energy is primarily stored as visceral fat, which we've learned causes inflammation in the body. You're also not using your muscles and benefitting from the anti-inflammatory myokines they release (see chapter 11), which adds to the pro-inflammatory state.

On average, people in the UK spend 9.5 hours per day sitting; as a nation we have a huge problem. Our lives change as we get older and most of us sit more. As runners, we tend to think that as long as we're running, we're active enough. Doing parkrun on a Saturday morning doesn't mean you can crash on the sofa for the rest of the day, because the exercise doesn't cancel out the sitting time – the risks are independent.

If you have a very active job and never get to sit down, you might be cursing it, but you'll be healthier than someone who is desk bound. But, what do you do when you aren't at work? Of course, we all need time to rest and recover, and I'm not suggesting that you shouldn't put your feet up from time to time. Simply check on yourself to make sure you are active on and off through every day, regardless of whether you're at work or not.

Being less sedentary is an easy win when it comes to improving our health. We can't just rely on our running. Notice your behaviour and make simple changes. For example:

- Use a sports watch or app to remind you to move every 30 to 60 minutes.
- Look at what you can do standing up that you usually do sitting down, such as working, making phone calls or being in an online meeting.
- Stand on public transport or stop frequently on long car journeys.
- Get up in the TV ad breaks.

Build up your standing time gradually to avoid back pain or other twinges. If you're working, make sure your desk and computer are at the right height to maintain a good posture. This book was written with my laptop on a box on my windowsill. Standing dead still is best avoided, but it's easy to rock, sway and do the odd stretch or squat while you're on your feet. Walking is even better than standing so try a walking work meeting or a take-away coffee with a friend. Stand on the train, get off a stop early and walk the rest of the way. I'm sure you get my drift!

These changes seem so small at the time, but with repetition day after day and week after week, they make a big difference. If you stand for 15 minutes extra per day, that works out as seven hours a month or three and a half days in a year. Imagine if you increased that to 30 minutes. Change can feel hard and overwhelming, but this is easy and embedding it into our everyday life will make a huge difference to our future health. Don't worry about sleeping, though. This is not the same as being sedentary. Sleep is a restorative state, and different from being inactive and awake, although don't sleep all the time!

> 'I run three to four times per week. My weight has stayed the same, but my waistline has changed from in my forties. I feel this is due to menopause.'
> **Jodi Clouston-Kerr**

HRT AND BODY COMPOSITION

One thing we can be pretty sure of is that HRT doesn't make you gain weight. For all the reasons we've discussed, weight is increasing anyway. HRT actually helps some women to lose weight, because they can move more freely, have more energy and be more motivated to exercise and make good food choices. What we can't be so sure of is the effect that HRT has on body composition. Some studies are indicating it may help to redistribute fat and reduce visceral fat. It may also have a positive effect on muscle growth, but the evidence isn't conclusive and the mechanisms aren't clear. These should certainly not be your primary reasons for using HRT.

ACTION STEPS

I hope you can see that regardless of your weight or shape, the reduction in muscle mass and the increase in visceral fat has the potential to negatively affect your long-term health. Now is the ideal opportunity to think about your body in terms of health over weight and make small, daily, lifestyle improvements. Here are the most important points:

1. There are no quick fixes. Close the door to anyone who says they have a magic remedy. This is about consistent changes to everyday behaviours. Expect improvement over months not weeks.
2. Reduce the amount of time you spend sitting to avoid your body going into storage mode.
3. Build your muscle mass through running and strength exercises.
4. Just eating less won't bring about the changes you seek and need.
5. Step away from the scales and find a better way to track your progress to good health. How your clothes fit and how you feel are perfect.

CHAPTER 13

Skin

Women tell me that alongside sagging and wrinkles in menopause, their skin becomes more delicate and sensitive. This can be challenging for runners. Blisters, chafing or skin irritation appear out of nowhere. A bright red face, hives and sweat rashes become common after a run. As runners our skin gets a hard time. It's regularly exposed to the elements, friction, sweat and to frequent washing, so we need to take care of it.

Skin is our biggest organ and it's incredible. It holds us together, keeps out water and germs, and makes vitamin D. It has a crucial role in regulating our body temperature. It grows as we grow, stretches, repairs itself and gives us the sensation of touch.

Skin is made of three layers. The epidermis is the outer layer. It's quite thin and contains pigment cells called melanocytes, which give it colour. Skin cells are constantly being shed at the surface and replaced by new cells, which mature as they move up through the epidermis. The next layer is called the dermis and it's much thicker. It contains sweat glands, hair follicles, blood vessels and nerve endings. Here you'll find a criss-cross of collagen fibres, which add structure and support, and elastic fibres, which allow stretch. Beneath the dermis is the hypodermis, a layer of subcutaneous fat which helps to cushion us, keep us warm and stores energy.

Skin reflects our general health and what's going on in our lives. Age, stress levels, nutrition and sun exposure all affect skin. So do our genetics, environment and exercise levels. It's even thought that in addition to our skin microbiome, the microbiome in our gut can impact skin health. We can't put all skin changes down to menopause, but skin is heavily influenced by hormones. Over time and with falling oestrogen levels, the collagen content and elasticity of skin reduces, the hypodermic layer shrinks and skin becomes drier. The epidermis becomes thinner and new cell production slows down. These changes lead to skin sagging, thinning and wrinkles. Sometimes hair follicles on the face become more active due to a change in the ratio of oestrogen and testosterone, leading to new growth of facial hair.

It's crucial to acknowledge all the factors that influence our skin health and not just blame menopause and age. There are lots of things we can do as menopausal runners to look after our skin and protect it for the future. Now is the perfect time to act.

SKIN CHAFING

Chafing can be intensely painful while you run and eye-wateringly sore in the shower afterwards! It happens when either skin or fabric rubs against skin. The skin cells at the top of the epidermis are rubbed away exposing cells which aren't yet mature enough to be at the outer layer. Nerve endings and blood vessels become exposed, which is why chafed skin can bleed and is so painful.

Most runners learn how to avoid chafing and it can come as a surprise when it starts becoming an issue again around menopause. One reason for this is increased sweating as the body tries to regulate its temperature; damp clothes and damp skin are a recipe for chafing disaster. The parts of your body that sweat and how much they sweat can alter with menopause. If your body shape is changing, your clothes may not fit like they used to. Chafing around sports bras that don't fit well, around short sleeves that have become a bit tight or between thighs are common problem areas. Finally, the reduced resiliency and plumpness of skin due to age and hormone changes means that skin is more vulnerable to damage and slower to heal.

Preventing chafed skin

Being aware that your skin may be more prone to getting chafed means you can take steps to prevent it. Here are some tips:

- Check your clothes fit well. Clothes that are too loose or too tight can cause issues.

- Get re-fitted for your sports bra. Breast size and shape can change in menopause.
- Choose technical fabrics. These wick sweat away from the body and dry quickly.
- Use a lubricant or barrier cream. Apply pre-run to problem areas such as around bra straps and inner thighs. If you sweat heavily or it's raining, try a nappy cream designed for babies, particularly around your bottom and perineum.
- Keep cool. For more about managing your body thermostat and reducing sweating, see chapter 3.
- Find a good antiperspirant. These won't directly protect your skin, but can reduce sweating by blocking pores. Be liberal with your use, but don't apply them near your vulva.
- Use moisturiser. Keep skin supple with regular moisturising. It doesn't have to be expensive. In fact, you'll probably use it more if you aren't counting the pennies with every smear.

Treating chafed skin

Despite our best efforts, chafing can happen. Even though it stings, give the skin a good wash with warm soapy water. Dry it thoroughly with a clean towel, as damp skin breeds germs. Apply Sudocrem or another cream containing zinc oxide, a mild antiseptic which creates a protective barrier. Leave the skin exposed to the air, but if you need to cover it up to prevent further rubbing, use a sterile dressing. Skin repair takes longer as we get older, so it might take a few days to heal. A mild itch and slight redness is normal, but it shouldn't get sticky or smelly and the redness should gradually reduce rather than spread. If these things happen, it indicates possible infection. Speak to your pharmacist about what you can buy over the counter and whether you need to see your doctor.

> ## GOOD TO KNOW
>
> Intertrigo is the name given to inflammation of skin in a skin fold, for example under breasts, in the groin or between the buttocks. The skin can get red, soggy and peel or crack. It's made worse by heat and sweat, so menopausal runners are a prime target for it. Intertrigo can commonly get infected with either bacteria or fungi, such as candida albicans (thrush). Treatment depends on the underlying cause, but follow the tips for chafed skin and speak to your pharmacist about which creams to use.

SKIN FLUSHING

My face gets redder than it ever used to after exercise and I have endless 'tomato face' selfies on my social media. The beetroot glow lasts for hours and it's easy to feel embarrassed by it. Lots of women tell me it puts them off exercise and they don't like the way it makes them look really unfit when they're not.

The body thermostat operates in a narrower range in perimenopause and the cooling mechanisms fire off much more frequently (see chapter 3). One of the ways the body cools itself is by widening the superficial blood vessels to increase blood flow to the skin. Blood that runs close to the surface of the skin can lose its heat more easily. Cooler blood returns to the body's core and lowers its temperature. The skin has a rich blood supply with a dense network of capillaries, and once these are expanded and full of blood the skin looks red.

Face flushing is caused by our autonomic nervous system, which we can't control. We can, however, keep cool and hydrated, not run during the hottest part of the day and generally avoid hot-flush triggers. On a positive note, a red face means that your body is effectively getting rid of excess heat and increased blood flow brings oxygen, healing cells and nutrients, and takes away toxins. How red you are is not a marker of how fit you are. Remember that other people probably won't even notice your red face and they're likely cheering you on rather than judging you.

Skin Sensitivity

Around one-third of women say their skin became more sensitive in peri- and post-menopause. Falling oestrogen and testosterone levels result in less skin oils (sebum) being produced. These oils help skin to retain moisture and less of them means skin dries out more quickly. You might develop skin sensitivities and rashes, particularly when you're hot and sweaty after a run. Heat and sweat rashes, hives and blotches are all common. Fluctuating oestrogen levels can affect the amount of histamine in the body which may contribute to the increased sensitivity of skin. Hormonal fluctuations, skin thinning and dryness all make the skin prone to itching (pruritis). For some this is intense. If you're really itchy, don't assume it's menopause. Your doctor may order blood tests to rule out liver, thyroid and kidney conditions. Coping with constantly dry, itchy and sensitive skin can be a real challenge. Here are some things you can try:

- Spot triggers. Keep a diary to help you find them. Alcohol, stress and certain foods might be exacerbating your skin condition.
- Keep your skin cool. For more about how to manage your body temperature, see chapter 3.
- Avoid really hot baths and showers which can dry out your skin and don't stay in too long.
- Use mild cleansers instead of soap and avoid strong or perfumed products.
- Keep skin hydrated and well moisturised. Moisturise within three minutes of washing when your skin is still damp, and on and off through the day, too. A high oil-content moisturiser will lock in more moisture. Don't skimp – use a thick layer. Give it a couple of minutes before you dress to let the skin absorb it.
- Apply a moisturiser to your face before you head out for a run, particularly on a windy day. Dab on some lip balm too.
- Speak to your pharmacist regarding anti-itch creams and anti-histamine medications.
- Adding oatmeal or baking soda to your bath water can help reduce itching.

- HRT can be beneficial if oestrogen levels are the main cause of skin symptoms and they're linked to flushes, sweats and disturbed sleep.

> 'I've started getting blotches and itchy lumps on my chest and neck after some of my runs. My skin just feels super-sensitive. It's really random and I can't work out what causes it.'
> **Anonymous**

GOOD TO KNOW

Dry and cracked skin on your feet can make running uncomfortable and you're more prone to infection as germs can creep into those cracks. A good tip is to apply a rich, oil-based moisturiser before bed and pop on some 100 per cent cotton socks. These will act like a dressing and help to retain moisture. Be warned though, some runners find super-soft skin on their feet makes them more likely to get blisters. It can be a fine balance!

SKIN SAGGING

It's inevitable that skin will sag a bit with age. How much is largely determined by skin elasticity, which is mainly down to your genetics. With age, the collagen content in the dermis reduces, so there is less skin structure and support. The fatty layer thins too, again reducing the support but also the plumpness of skin. You might notice that your cheeks are hollower and the skin under your chin is looser. Some people will blame running for these changes and call it 'runner's face', but it's important to know that running is not the reason. Lifestyle does influence skin sagging, but that is down to sun exposure, nutrition and hydration, not the up and down movement of running. The rest is down to genetics. Regular exercise is really important for healthy-looking skin.

> ### GOOD TO KNOW
>
> Women over 50 struggle with dry eye disease twice as much as men. Eyes can feel sore, gritty and irritated. They can itch and crust and you can become intolerant of contact lenses. It's thought that reducing hormone levels in menopause affect the meibomian glands which sit along the lash line and secrete an oily substance called meibum onto the surface of the eye. Meibum traps watery tears and reduces the speed they evaporate away. We produce less meibum and fewer tears as we get older, too. If your eyes water excessively when you run this may actually be down to dry eyes. Tear production increases to counteract hot, cold or windy weather, all of which can dry out eyes. Reducing your screen time, using artificial tear drops and wearing glasses when you run can all help.

SUN DAMAGE

One of the most important ways we can look after our skin is to limit exposure to the harmful UV rays of the sun and know how to spot the signs of sun damage. As runners we're outside a lot, often for long periods of time and in direct sunlight, and we need to be much more vigilant about our skin than most people.

Sunburn

Your skin may burn more easily than it ever used to. This is partly due to a fall in the number and activity of melanocytes in the dermis layer of your skin. Melanocytes produce melanin, which is skin pigment, and they send it out to the skin cells at the outermost layer of the skin, in little round packages called melanosomes. The melanosomes position themselves above the nuclei of these cells to protect them, and the DNA contained within them, from UV radiation. I like to think of this as little sun shades for the nuclei. Oestrogen seems to have a role in regulating melanin production. Fluctuating oestrogen levels can alter skin pigment and affect the amount of melanin produced and therefore the ability of the skin to protect itself from the sun. Higher levels of melanin can cause age spots. Lower levels result in fewer sun shades to go around and they become flimsier, and don't give such good shade. The reduced thickness of skin that happens with age and falling oestrogen levels can also contribute to an increased risk of sunburn.

Regardless of your skin shade, you can still get sunburn. You're less likely to get burned if you have black or brown skin, and the risk of skin cancer is lower, but it isn't zero. Intermittently burning is worse for your skin than gradual tanning. If you've never given much consideration to protecting your skin, other than the odd dollop of sunscreen on a hot day, now is absolutely the time to do it. Both menopause and ageing mean our skin is more at risk of damage and action now will pay off in the future.

Actinic keratoses

These dry, rough or scaly skin lesions are more common over age 50. They're also known as solar keratoses, because they're related to many years of sun exposure. They're about 1 to 2 centimetres in size and are usually found on the face, forearms, head and legs, in areas which see the most sun. They can be a range of colours, from your normal skin colour through to pink and red. An actinic keratosis will usually go away on its own, but there is a small risk it can turn into a squamous cell carcinoma, a form of skin cancer, so it's best removed. This can be done using creams and gels, freezing treatments or surgery to scrape it away or cut it out.

Basal cell carcinoma

Basal cell carcinoma (BCC) is a type of skin cancer which is related to sun exposure. Basal cells are found at the bottom of the epidermis and they make the new skin cells which gradually move to the surface of the skin. Changes in the DNA of the cell cause it to become abnormal and over-multiply. Like actinic keratoses, BCCs usually develop on sun-exposed skin, but they can crop up anywhere. They vary in their appearance, but they're usually a raised lump of some sort which grows slowly over time. BCCs may look transparent, but on white skin they can look pink and on brown or black skin they can be dark brown or black. The outside border of the lesion is often raised and they sometimes bleed or crust over. Unlike melanoma, it's very rare for a BCC to spread to other parts of your body or to cause you any harm. They can be fully removed with surgery.

Malignant melanoma

Melanoma is a type of skin cancer and it's becoming more common every year. Cancer Research UK say that 86 per cent of melanomas are preventable. The main cause of melanoma is UV light from the sun and sunbeds, which damages the DNA of the melanocyte cells in the skin and causes them to multiply uncontrollably. Melanoma can metastasise (spread) to other parts of the body, so it's vital to identify and treat it early. We're all at risk of melanoma, but that risk grows as we get older. It's also higher if we have pale skin, lots of moles or a family history of skin cancer. Again, sun-exposed skin is the most likely area for a melanoma, but if you have black or brown skin, then be alert for black lesions under nails or on the soles of your feet and palms of your hands.

GOOD TO KNOW

Melanomas can also occur in the eye. While the exact cause of ocular melanomas is unclear and many happen by chance, exposure to UV radiation is thought to be a risk factor. Eyelashes provide some protection from the sun but many women find their lashes become thinner and sparser during menopause. A decent pair of running sunglasses which block out UV rays is a wise investment.

> ### When should I go to the doctor?
>
> Keep a close eye on your skin and watch for new lesions or changes in existing ones. Most skin rashes, lumps and bumps are not skin cancer, but it's best to get anything unusual checked out. See your doctor if:
>
> - You have a mole that is:
>   - growing in size or thickness
>   - bleeding, crusted or inflamed
>   - itchy
>   - changing colour, getting darker or speckled becoming irregular, uneven or spreading outwards into the surrounding skin.
> - You have a skin lesion that has been present for a few weeks and you don't know what it is.

PROTECTING YOUR SKIN FROM THE SUN

Being a runner in peri- or post-menopause puts us at more risk of sun damage to our skin. We need to take action and there are simple steps that make a difference. Keeping out of the sun is an obvious one – that might mean not running in the middle of the day during summer or choosing shady routes. You can check the UV index on local weather forecasts and apps, and the higher the number, the more risk there is of the sun causing damage. For most skin types, a UV index above 3 indicates risk and you should take steps to protect your skin.

Wear a sunscreen with at least SPF 15 whenever you run, even on cloudy days. Find a sunscreen that doesn't slide into your eyes when you sweat and make them sting. Covering up is simple yet effective, so if you're on a long run, then a vest top probably isn't the best option. If your body thermostat can take it, opt for a light t-shirt, ideally with long sleeves. Put your face in the shade with a cap or visor. Some have flaps on the back to cover your neck too. Remember, this is something we can control and good habits improve our future skin health.

GOOD TO KNOW

Long-term skin conditions such as eczema, psoriasis and rosacea can be unpredictable in menopause. You may find you get flare-ups of your condition due to hormonal fluctuations, and the changing structure and integrity of skin. If this is happening to you, see your doctor to discuss your treatment. You may just need to be more diligent in your skin care and avoid triggers or you may need a step up in any medications you use.

SKIN AGEING

If this chapter is making you feel that as a runner your skin is doomed and you're worrying about premature skin ageing as a result, then relax. We definitely need to take extra steps to protect our skin, but running is not going to make us look older. Remember that so many factors affect our skin, not just menopause and not just being outside more than the average person. Exercise itself is anti-ageing. Chromosomes which store our genetic material have little protective caps on the end of them called telomeres. As you get older and as cells are damaged from oxidative stress building up inside them, the telomeres shorten. This eventually exposes the DNA and cell damage or early cell death can occur. We know that regular exercise helps to prevent oxidative stress in cells, which means that telomere shortening is slowed down, and less early cell death and damage occurs. The result is the anti-ageing effect of exercise. Keep running, but don't forget your sunscreen.

'My skin has become even drier, less elastic and more papery in perimenopause. It looks like it's dropping off my face and I have little fine lines on my chin. On the plus side, I have no break-outs and there's nothing some good retinol at night and vitamin C serum in the morning doesn't 'zhuzh up'!'

Sue Reynolds, Harrogate

CHAPTER 14

Mental Health

Mental health symptoms can be the first sign that you're perimenopausal and can affect you as much as, if not more than, physical symptoms. Sometimes mental health problems come as a result of physical symptoms. In the Moving Through Menopause report by Scottish Action for Mental Health (SAMH), more than 60 per cent of respondents indicated that a menopause symptom had a negative impact on their mental well-being. That level rose to 80 per cent for the symptoms of mood, brain fog and sleep disturbance (that wasn't due to night sweats). Most runners tell me they didn't start running for mental health reasons, but they're the main reason they continue with running in menopause, helping them to regulate their mood, cope with stress and take time for themselves.

HOW DOES MENOPAUSE AFFECT MENTAL HEALTH?

There are a wide range of mental health symptoms you might experience, including:

- Mood swings
- Irritability
- Anger
- Feeling antisocial
- Difficulty concentrating
- Brain fog
- Poor memory
- Irrational fears
- Panic attacks

- Anxiety
- Depression
- Loss of motivation
- Loss of competitive drive
- Loss of identity
- Loss of confidence
- Poor self-esteem
- Not feeling in control.

If you have mental health problems that pre-exist your perimenopause, they may or may not get worse during menopause. If you've had hormonal mood changes in the past, for example post-natal depression, premenstrual syndrome (PMS) or premenstrual dysphoric disorder (PMDD), then you will be at higher risk of mood changes during menopause, but the more even hormonal pattern in post-menopause will bring more stable moods. The link between hormone shifts and mood disorders is emerging and needs more research and study. Being aware of the possibility of an increased risk of mental health conditions means you can be prepared, look out for signs and take early action.

GOOD TO KNOW

Recent research has shown a significantly increased rate of women developing bipolar disorder for the first time during perimenopause. It's not clear yet whether this is directly linked to perimenopause or to this age and stage of life more generally, but it drops again in post-menopause, suggesting it is hormonally driven.

RUNNING AND MENTAL HEALTH SYMPTOMS

Mental health symptoms can have an impact on your desire and ability to run. If you're feeling antisocial, you might skip running club. If you've developed an irrational fear, such as a fear of motorway driving, you might stop going to races. Anxiety and panic attacks can make you nervous to run alone, even on your favourite routes. Brain fog and inability to concentrate make route planning difficult. Loss of motivation is a big problem, too – getting yourself out the door on a wet evening when you're tired is hard enough without any additional hormonal lack of enthusiasm.

Many women find that they lose the desire to compete or really challenge themselves. This can be a big issue if competition, whether it be against others or yourself, is a major motivator for you to train. This loss of competitive drive may be due to reducing levels of testosterone as this hormone has been linked to competitiveness in men. However, there is a lack of studies looking at testosterone effects in women. There is evidence that oestrogen is linked to competitiveness, too, so the hormones may act differently in the different sexes. As is often the case with menopause, it's probably a combination of factors. Of course, a declining performance can reduce your competitive drive, too, because not getting the results you want can be very demotivating and make you less inclined to compete.

Running can be a huge part of our identity. It's what we do. We're 'runners' and others perceive us that way too. If menopause makes running really hard for you, you might run less, feel ashamed of how you're running and ultimately struggle to call yourself a runner. With all the changes that go on in menopause, a loss of identity is very common. You might not recognise yourself physically and you might be acting in ways that are unusual for you, flying off the handle or crying easily. When I was working as a GP, I remember women coming to me and saying, 'I just don't recognise myself any more, I don't know who I am.' Your thoughts, feelings and appearance can all be affected. Adding the loss of identity as a runner to this mix can amplify these changes. If you feel like this, you are not alone and it will pass. You are still you, but it takes time and patience to find yourself again.

'Running to improve my mental health during perimenopause has become my go-to reason to run. The anxiety has been crippling at times, but running really helps.'
Emma Davies, South Wales

WHY DOES MENOPAUSE AFFECT MENTAL HEALTH?

It's important to consider the bigger picture and all that's going on in the lives of women at this stage of life, because this massively affects how we feel mentally:

Getting older: Natural signs of ageing appear, such as greying hair, wrinkles and generally feeling older. Many women struggle with the concept of ageing for multiple reasons, including feeling less beautiful, less feminine and less relevant.

Loss of fertility: We may have mixed reactions to our child-bearing years coming to an end. There could be relief, but also great sadness.

Family changes: You may be facing an empty nest or the loss of or ageing parents. If you started your family over 40 or have an early or premature menopause, it may coincide with children starting primary or secondary school. In the UK in 2024, the average age for women to be divorced was 44, which is during perimenopause for many women.

Career changes: You may be in a senior leadership position and at the peak of your career. On the other hand, you may be starting over in a new direction.

Poor sleep: Sleep can be worse with hormonal changes, symptoms of menopause and with stress from all of the above.

Every woman is different and how every woman feels, approaches and experiences these life events will vary hugely. There's no doubt, though, that there are significant events going on in the lives of women at the very time that menopause strikes and the combination of the two can have a huge effect on mental health.

> 'I'm far less able to manage stress and this decreases my energy levels much further. With everything women have to juggle, it's not surprising we feel burnout when going through menopause.'
> **Sarah**

BRAIN CHANGES IN MENOPAUSE

The menopausal brain is currently a hot topic for researchers. The fluctuations and decline in oestrogen, progesterone and testosterone have direct effects on brain function. Our brain is changing and remodelling as it adapts to a new phase of life.

A study from 2021 showed that as the women studied moved from peri- to post-menopause, there were changes in brain structure, the way different areas of the brain connected with each other and in the way the brain used energy. These changes did not occur in men, so were not simply related to ageing. Thankfully this study also showed that many of the changes are transient, for example an area of the brain that involves memory reduces in volume during perimenopause but the brain responds, increases energy production and blood flow in this area, and it recovers in post-menopause. Different parts of the brain are responsible for thoughts, feelings and actions, so changes in these will lead to specific symptoms.

Studies have shown that the density of oestrogen receptors in the brain increases as you move into post-menopause, particularly in areas of the brain where you're getting symptoms. The brain adapts and wants to make the most of the oestrogen available so it ramps up the number of receptors oestrogen can bind to in certain areas of the brain.

Oestrogen is sometimes known as a 'happy hormone' and progesterone as a 'calming hormone'. They undoubtedly have direct effects on how we feel, but we know that they also influence other powerful mood modulators in the brain, such as dopamine, serotonin, cortisol, endorphins and melatonin, which all play a role in our mood, stress and anxiety levels. It's a complex and largely poorly understood network of communication between different areas of the brain, and different hormones and neurotransmitters. Oestrogen seems to play a much more pivotal role in this than we have previously given it credit for.

CORTISOL AND STRESS

Cortisol is a stress hormone which naturally ebbs and flows according to our circadian rhythms and what's going on in our lives. Cortisol is made in the adrenal glands, which sit just above the kidneys. Levels rise in the morning, helping us to feel awake, and reduce at night to aid sleep. When we're under stress, levels of cortisol are higher. That's handy for short-term stressful events as it helps us to perform well, but if we're under chronic (long-term) stress, it's a different story. High levels of cortisol for months on end can have a negative effect on our health, causing weight gain, high blood pressure and mood changes. Many women have become afraid of high-intensity exercise due to fear of raising their cortisol levels even higher. Those short, sharp bursts of cortisol are not the problem and they're very different to the longer, grumbling, raised cortisol linked to chronic stress (see chapter 12).

CHICKEN OR EGG?

For many women, the symptoms of menopause are the cause of their mental health problems. If hot flushes and brain fog make you unable to do your job properly, and muscle aches and breast tenderness make running hard, your stress levels can increase and your mood can drop. Not having running as your coping mechanism can cause anxiety levels to rise. Anxiety and depression are well known to cause sleep disturbance and being sleep deprived undoubtedly makes these conditions worse. It's a vicious circle to be caught in. While there may not be an easy solution, it's worth understanding that cause and effect are entwined when it comes to mental health. Take a step back, look at the bigger picture and control the things you can control.

> 'I have anxious moments from time to time and I really notice my grumpy mood when I haven't been able to get out and run.'
> **Jodi Clouston-Kerr**

ANXIETY AND MENOPAUSE

Going into a job interview or lining up for a long-trained-for race will almost certainly make you feel anxious. Your body's response can help you to focus and perform well. When anxiety happens without a trigger and doesn't ease off, then you're stepping into the realm of anxiety disorders. There are many different types of anxiety, ranging from panic attacks to generalised anxiety disorder (GAD).

Anxiety is often the first perimenopausal symptom that women experience. A study from 2013 found that women who had low levels of anxiety in pre-menopause were more likely to report high anxiety levels in the early and late perimenopause and in post-menopause, too. However, those who already had anxiety in pre-menopause continued with high levels of anxiety unrelated to their stage of menopause. Anxiety can have a big effect on your running. You might experience:

- A lack of belief in your ability.
- Feeling overwhelmed by a training plan.
- Fear about the logistics of getting to an event.
- Fatigue and poor recovery from lack of sleep and the energy that worrying uses.
- An elevated heart rate.
- Increased gastrointestinal problems.
- Severe pre-race nerves.

Anxiety can seem to come out of nowhere and knock you off your feet. You can feel it physically as well as mentally: palpitations, nausea and shakiness are common. A constant feeling of being on edge, jittery or hyper alert is exhausting and upsetting.

> 'I'm crabby, irritable and short with my family. I cry a lot. I work full-time, am a wife, mom and a friend. As a social worker, my job requires listening to others' problems and having to absorb their issues. I love what I do and my patients. There are times when I sit in my office and cry, sometimes for no reason at all. I'm on medication for depression and anxiety, and I see a counsellor. But it's a lot some days.'
> **Carri Ables**

Depression and Menopause

The brain is going through a lot of change during the menopause transition, making us vulnerable and more at risk of mental health conditions such as depression. A 2024 study of over 9000 women found that women were around 40 per cent more likely to develop depression in perimenopause than they were to develop it before they had any menopausal symptoms. However, researchers didn't find an increased risk of developing depression in post-menopause compared to life before perimenopause. It makes sense that during that peri phase, when symptoms are at their greatest, we might be at our most vulnerable.

The symptoms of depression and menopause overlap and it can be hard to know whether you're experiencing depression or the psychological symptoms of menopause. If you're depressed, your sleep can be disturbed, your energy can be low and you can find it very hard to focus and concentrate. You might have no sex drive, lose your appetite and feel very down and negative. All of these things can happen in menopause, too. Distinguishing between depression and the mood disorders of menopause is important, though, because the treatments are different.

Being depressed makes running really hard. A lack of enjoyment of the things that used to bring you pleasure is a common symptom of depression. It's called anhedonia. Couple that with low motivation and fatigue from sleep problems and it's easy to see why your running can be severely affected. Even when you know it will do you good, it's difficult to do.

> ### When to see your doctor
> Mental health is just as important as physical health, yet there's still a hesitancy to talk about it. Don't see making a doctor's appointment as a failure or last resort. Don't let yourself get to rock bottom before you ask for help. See your doctor if:
>
> - You have symptoms of depression or anxiety that are affecting your ability to work, care for your family or live your normal daily life.

- You have any thoughts of hurting or harming yourself in any way.
- You experience unusual symptoms, such as hearing voices, seeing things that aren't really there or you have a sense that someone or something is watching you, controlling you or influencing you in some way.
- You have episodes or a constant feeling of extreme elation, racing thoughts or extreme changes in mood.
- You've tried self-help steps, but aren't feeling any better.
- Your symptoms of depression aren't improving despite being on treatments such as hormone therapy or antidepressants.

BRAIN FOG

Brain fog, the feeling that your head is full of cotton wool, is often laughed about, but it can be devastating. Around two-thirds of women in menopause experience it, and it's frustrating, inconvenient and can make you feel silly and lose your confidence. The biggest impact is often felt at work. Forgetting names and important information, going blank and having to constantly make lists of what you need to do are common symptoms. One study found that one in 10 women had left a job, 14 per cent had reduced their hours and 8 per cent had not applied for a promotion because of menopause symptoms.

Resolving brain fog is not easy. The most important thing to know is that it's temporary and it will go. It's not a sign that you are going to develop dementia. You are not any less intelligent because you have brain fog. Some but not all women find that HRT helps their brain fog clear, particularly if it improves their sleep. Healthy lifestyle changes, particularly improving your sleep, can often help to ease brain fog.

> ### GOOD TO KNOW
>
> Alzheimer's disease is the commonest form of dementia. Two-thirds of people with Alzheimer's disease are women, partly because women live longer. Declining memory and thinking (cognitive function) are in part due to plaques and tangles of amyloid and tau, two proteins which build up in the brain and stop it working properly. There are lots of risk factors that increase your likelihood of developing Alzheimer's disease but age, sex and genetics are the most important and the ones we can't change. What we can control, however, is our lifestyle, and keeping physically, mentally and socially active all help to reduce our risk. Regular exercise can reduce the risk by 20 per cent and maintaining physical activity through midlife is particularly beneficial.

MIGRAINE AND MENOPAUSE

While not a mental health condition, migraine affects the brain, can be influenced by how you're feeling mentally and can also determine your mental state. People who have migraine have a four times higher risk of anxiety than those who do not have migraine. Migraine can cause anxiety, but anxiety can cause migraine! We really need to talk about it, because three times as many women have migraine than men and it can start or worsen in perimenopause. Migraine attacks can generally become more frequent and difficult to manage in menopause. They can put you out of action for a few days at a time and have a significant impact on your daily life, including your ability to run.

Migraine is not purely about headaches. In fact, some people who have migraine don't get a headache with it at all. Other symptoms include nausea, vomiting and dizziness. Altered vision, light sensitivity and brain fog are common, too.

We don't understand why but the brain of people with migraine tends to be more sensitive to change. That change might be external, including disturbed sleep, stress or even the weather. It can also be internal, such as hydration, blood sugar levels or hormonal fluctuations. During menopause, there is a lot of change going on and hormonal fluctuations, disturbed sleep and stress are all common. This explains why migraine attacks can become more frequent.

Some women find that exercise can be a trigger for migraine, particularly if it's sudden, high-intensity exercise. Research has shown that exercising at a mild or moderate intensity three times a week for half an hour can help to reduce migraine attacks. Regular strength training and yoga (avoiding head down positions and abrupt changes in posture) have both been shown to be beneficial, too.

In terms of medication, it's key to get the right treatment at the right time and treat attacks early to prevent them building up. Speak to your doctor about what to use when. If your migraine is not controlled, you can be referred to a headache specialist or book directly with the National Migraine Centre if you are in the UK.

When it comes to lifestyle, it's all about minimising change. Establishing routines and eating regularly can help. Spend time warming up rather than abruptly starting to run. Drink plenty of fluids and fuel your runs well to keep your hydration and blood sugar levels even (see chapter 16). Make sure you run with good posture to avoid strain on your neck and shoulders, which can trigger migraine in some people. If your stress levels are high, reducing them may improve your migraine, but it may not and it can be hard to do! Sometimes smoothing out hormonal fluctuations using contraceptive pills or HRT can be beneficial, so speak to your doctor about this, especially if self-care steps aren't working.

LIFESTYLE STEPS FOR MENTAL HEALTH SYMPTOMS IN MENOPAUSE

Lifestyle changes are important for all of us, both to maintain good mental health, but also to help us cope when we're not feeling good. I'll say it again: control what you can control:

- **Reduce your stress levels:** Easier said than done, but it's crucial to try. You may need to be assertive and brave to do this. In all your roles, identify what you can give up, delegate or change. Be realistic about what you can cope with and be the best advocate for yourself.

- **Maximise your nutrition:** Reduce caffeine and alcohol – this can reduce feelings of jitteriness and anxiety as well as improve sleep and lift mood – and eat well and regularly. Avoid the ups and downs of a sugar rollercoaster (see chapter 16).
- **Connect with others:** Talk to someone you trust. Good social health improves mental health so find people or communities where you can relax, be yourself and have a sense of belonging.
- **Make time to laugh:** This is hard when you feel depressed, but laughter helps with stress reduction, learning and well-being.
- **Celebrate good things:** Challenge your negative thoughts and celebrate any small wins you can find.
- **Improve your sleep:** It can be hard to do, but any steps you take to prioritise your sleep will help improve your mental health (see chapter 4).

MEDICAL TREATMENTS FOR MENTAL HEALTH SYMPTOMS IN MENOPAUSE

The first-line treatment for the mood changes of menopause is HRT, it is not antidepressants. This is where a good discussion with your doctor is needed to see if you can unpick whether you have depression as a medical condition or the psychological symptoms of menopause. Using an antidepressant hasn't been shown to help mood changes related to menopause if you don't have a diagnosis of depression. For more about hormone therapy, see chapter 15.

Cognitive behavioural therapy (CBT) is also extremely useful. With or without HRT or antidepressants, this talking therapy challenges the way you think, feel and behave. Identifying and stopping unhelpful thinking patterns can help you feel better and find other ways to deal with problems.

There are a variety of medications used to help resolve both anxiety and depression. For example, low doses of beta-blockers can help to reduce anxiety and palpitations. Some mood-changing medications used for depression also have other beneficial effects when it comes to menopause (see chapter 15). We are all different and how we each tolerate and respond to medications varies hugely, too. It may take some trial and error and multiple visits to the doctor, but never feel as if you are being a pain in the neck. Your doctor wants to help you and there are always options.

> 'I am happier now that menopause is way in the past as my mood is more constant.'
> **Maggie Lightfoot**

HOW RUNNING HELPS MENTAL HEALTH IN MENOPAUSE

Look at the lifestyle steps for mental health symptoms on page 154 and notice how running helps with all of these, even nutrition, because running regularly can give you an increased interest in how you fuel your body.

Running can help you reduce stress, because it increases endorphin levels. These are the body's own happy hormones and they bind to the same brain receptors as opiates, which include drugs like morphine. Running also triggers the release of endocannabinoids, which are essentially the body's own cannabis, giving a feeling of euphoria, peace and reduced pain. Being able to trigger the release of such powerful anti-anxiety chemicals as and when you need them can be a real blessing in perimenopause. Running also benefits sleep (see chapter 4).

Whether you're feeling anxious, depressed or stressed, running can help you feel more in control. You can set and achieve goals to feel more positive and build your self-confidence. It also takes you into nature, which is known to have a calming effect, and the thud of your feet on the ground provides a meditative milieu to quieten your mind.

Running can help you to connect with others, from a knowing nod from a passing runner to a whole running community. Find running friends who understand the challenges and can support you to keep running. Your running community can help you to relax, laugh and to celebrate success. The barriers to running in menopause are huge, but the benefits to your mental health are bigger. Even if it's a short, easy walk outside, something is definitely better than nothing.

> 'Menopause for me can mean starting a day feeling any combination of groggy, irritable or anxious. However hard it is to get out for a run, I always feel so much better afterwards. Running has been a game-changer for me in these later years of perimenopause and into post-menopause. It's helped so much to restore a sense of balance and calm in my life.'
>
> **Helen L,** Lancaster

CHAPTER 15

Menopause Treatments

The good news is that there is so much we can do to help us get through this transition and smooth out the menopause rollercoaster. Running itself can be a wonderful treatment, but sometimes other treatments are needed in order for you to feel able to run. The bad news is that there are a lot of people making a lot of money out of the fact that we are, sometimes desperately, searching for answers and solutions. It's very easy to be drawn into cleverly designed marketing ploys. Being properly evidence-based is generally not trendy. It doesn't create clickbait headlines or eye-catching reels, but it is sound and safe. We all deserve to be treated in the correct way, based on high-quality, non-biased, huge randomised controlled trials and meta-analyses involving thousands of women, carried out by authors who don't have conflicts of interest.

LIFESTYLE AS TREATMENT

Think of lifestyle changes as your number one prescription. A healthy lifestyle includes good nutrition, sleep and stress reduction and it definitely includes running. Just as you would take a medication or supplement regularly, you need to take positive lifestyle steps consistently, every day. Give lifestyle the same priority as you would a prescribed medication. Don't think of it as the add-on, rather the foundation on which everything else is built.

HORMONE REPLACEMENT THERAPY

Hormone replacement therapy (HRT), increasingly known as menopause hormone therapy (MHT), is the main medical treatment for menopause. It can be a complicated and nuanced topic, but I want to give you a quick, no-nonsense guide that relates to you as a runner. I'm very grateful to Dr Cath Munro, who is a GP and an advanced British Menopause Society specialist, for her guidance and input into this chapter.

The key thing to remember is that every woman is different and HRT prescribing needs to be based on an individual's risks, benefits and preferences. You need a discussion with a doctor who can help you make the best decision for you, based on your medical history and current guidelines. This might be your GP or a GP in the practice with a special interest in menopause. It might be after referral to a local menopause clinic or via a menopause specialist in a private clinic.

Prescriptions for HRT are rising. In England in 2023, the number of women given a prescription rose by 12 per cent, compared to the previous 12-month period. However, total figures are low and only 15 per cent of women age 45 to 64 take HRT. This reflects women's perception of HRT and an inequality in access to it. In the least deprived areas of England, there are more than twice as many women using HRT compared to the most deprived areas. The figures also reflect a lack of knowledge and expertise within the medical profession, which is thankfully improving all the time.

HRT is definitely not a panacea for menopause. It can be life-changing for some women, but it should always be one part of the jigsaw and it should never be a replacement for healthy lifestyle changes, just an addition to them.

Who needs HRT?

There are several situations when you should consider HRT:

- You have an early or premature menopause – premature ovarian insufficiency (POI).
- You have menopause symptoms that are affecting your daily life.
- You have or are at high risk of developing osteoporosis.

There is not currently enough evidence to support giving HRT solely to prevent coronary heart disease, Alzheimer's disease, colorectal cancer or type 2 diabetes. These potential benefits may be part of your personal case that builds as all your risks and benefits are discussed, but should not be the sole factor that determines whether you take it or not.

> 'Some friends feel being unwell is inevitable and just get on with it. I went on HRT. Why should I put up with the symptoms when there are things that I can do to help? I've learned to swim and completed two half Ironman triathlons since going through menopause. Having a positive, can-do attitude helps me.'
> **Nikki Carpenter**

Who doesn't need HRT?

Not all women can or want to take HRT. If you've had an early or premature menopause and don't have a contraindication to HRT, then you are advised to take it up until at least age 51, the average age of menopause. Without it, you will have many added years of lower levels of oestrogen and that has long-term consequences, particularly when it comes to bone health.

If your menopause is around the average age, symptoms are manageable and there are no concerns about your bone health, you shouldn't feel any pressure to take HRT. You won't automatically end up a weak, shrivelled old lady in a matter of years without it. You can have a long, healthy and happy life without HRT.

> 'I chose not to use it. I didn't think my symptoms were so bad. Also I saw my mother have a bad reaction to HRT and when I was younger I had depression and anxiety from birth control pills so I had a fear of having a bad response to HRT.'
> **Colette,** Lancaster

Who can't take HRT?

HRT is safe for the vast majority of women. There are situations when it's not advised and these are mainly linked to conditions that are hormonally driven and where giving hormones could exacerbate or trigger them, such as with active breast cancer. Never assume you can or can't take HRT without a discussion with your doctor. They should liaise with any specialists who are also involved with your care and may refer you on to a menopause specialist.

Remember, there are treatments other than HRT to help ease menopausal symptoms. They're not generally as effective as HRT, but using them alongside lifestyle changes gives you options.

What symptoms will HRT improve?

Controlling symptoms is the main reason to take HRT and it's very effective at reducing the following symptoms in most women:

- Hot flushes.
- Night sweats.
- Sleep disturbance due to the above.
- Depressive symptoms of menopause.
- Genitourinary symptoms.

What symptoms will HRT not improve?

Generally, if a symptom is directly due to a lack of oestrogen or progesterone, then increasing the levels of those through using HRT will improve it. The problem is, it's common to put symptoms down to menopause and then get disappointed when HRT doesn't work. For example, if your anxiety is caused by a really stressful work life and a parent with dementia, then HRT is not going to help. If, however, your anxiety is caused by sleep deprivation from night sweats and poor work performance due to hot flushes, then HRT will be likely to reduce your anxiety. If your low mood is a direct result of hormonal changes, then HRT will be beneficial, but if it's due to bereavement or youngsters flying the nest, then your expectations should be realistic. Again, every woman is different and there can be overlapping causes; it's often a case of try it and see. You need at least three months on HRT before you really know how it's going to benefit you and to let any initial side-effects settle.

> 'My friend told me to arm myself with all the information I could and visit my GP. I did and got prescribed exactly the HRT that I asked for. My life changed. My hot flushes completely vanished and it's dampened other symptoms down to a level where I can cope. I'm happy again and no longer riddled with anxiety or constant heart palpitations. I was able to start running again!'
>
> **Sarah Jones,** Isle of Wight

When should I start taking HRT?

Taking HRT shouldn't be seen as a sign of failure and something you have to resort to when you're at your wits' end. You don't have to grin and bear it for as long as possible. Every woman is affected differently by menopause and the level of symptoms that feel acceptable to you will vary according to your work and home life, and even your cultural norms.

You can start HRT whenever you need to, whenever your symptoms are intrusive into your life. It's a myth that you can't take HRT while you're still having periods, you can. The greatest evidence of benefit from HRT is in women under 60. That doesn't mean you can't start it if you're over 60, but the risks and benefits for each individual woman have to be weighed up. Remember that if you have an early or premature menopause you will be advised to start using HRT as soon as the diagnosis is made. There are so many factors that need to be considered when it comes to prescribing HRT, it is really both an art and a science. Doses often need to be tweaked and changed over time, because you'll be changing and your HRT may need to as well.

When should I stop taking HRT?

You should stop HRT whenever the risks outweigh the benefits and of course at any point in between if you simply don't want to continue it. That risk/benefit balance varies hugely between women and it changes with time. This is why you should have an annual HRT review with your practice nurse or GP, to check whether any new conditions have arisen that might increase your risk and to assess how much it's helping you. Risks generally increase with age and length of time using HRT, but there is no arbitrary time limit and there are women in their eighties still using HRT. When it comes to stopping it, many women prefer to titrate down gradually. This might reduce the likelihood of symptoms coming back in the short term and can help to build confidence that you're going to be okay without it, but it's also fine to stop it abruptly.

What type of HRT do I need?

If you don't have a uterus, for example if you've had a hysterectomy, then you only need to use oestrogen. If you still have a uterus, then you need both oestrogen and a progestogen. Progestogens protect the endometrium, which is the lining of the uterus. Taking oestrogen without a progestogen or without sufficient progestogen for the dose of oestrogen you are taking can increase the risk of irregular bleeding, endometrial thickening and endometrial cancer.

You can choose to take oestrogen as a tablet, gel, patch or spray. You can have progestogen as a tablet, through the skin or via an intrauterine system (IUS), which is a coil that slowly releases synthetic progestogen into the uterus.

There are different types of oestrogen and the one most commonly used in HRT is 17-beta oestradiol. This is a 'body identical' oestrogen which means it has the same molecular structure as your own oestrogen.

Synthetic progestogens mimic the behaviour of the body's natural progesterone. They were originally developed because progesterone couldn't be absorbed orally. You might hear them referred to as progestins. Synthetic progestogens are not 'body identical' but there is now a 'body identical', micronized progesterone table available called Utrogestan™, which may be superior to using synthetic progestogen as part of HRT.

> ## GOOD TO KNOW
> Body identical and bioidentical hormones are not the same thing. Body identical hormones such as oestradiol or micronised progesterone are regulated and licensed medications. Bioidentical hormones are often sold as 'natural supplements'. They are unregulated, compounded products which means the ingredients are customised to individual women. The problem is that the hormone tests they are based on are often not accurate and the products haven't gone through the same rigorous trials, safety tests or quality controls that regulated medications go through. Your doctor cannot prescribe bioidentical compounded hormones and they aren't recommended by the British Menopause Society.

HRT absorbed through the skin goes straight into the bloodstream and gives a steadier level of hormones which can lead to better symptom control. If you're someone who has difficulty absorbing oestrogen tablets due to a gastrointestinal condition, then it can bypass that entirely. This route also reduces the risk of deep vein thrombosis (DVT) or pulmonary embolism (PE) and it can be used in women who take medications that affect liver enzymes. It's also the recommended way to take HRT if you have migraine, gall bladder disease or a BMI over 30.

If you have a uterus, are still having periods or are within 12 months of the last one when you first start taking HRT, you will be offered sequential therapy. This involves taking oestrogen every day and using progestogen for part of each 28-day cycle. It's usually taken for between 10 and 14 days of the cycle and you'll get a withdrawal bleed at the end of those days.

If you have a uterus and haven't had a period for a year or more (so you're post-menopausal) or you've been using cyclical HRT for over a year, then you may be offered continuous combined therapy which is a steady, daily dose of oestrogen and progestogen. This is often called 'no bleed HRT' because after six months of treatment you shouldn't have any bleeding.

> ### GOOD TO KNOW
>
> It's really important to see a doctor if you experience any bleeding from your vagina once you are post-menopausal. You should also see your doctor if you bleed for more than six months after starting continuous combined HRT or you've been taking it without having any bleeding and then suddenly you bleed. You will be referred for investigation to rule out endometrial cancer. Most women don't have endometrial cancer, but it's important to exclude it. Don't just wait to see if it settles down.

What are the risks of taking HRT?

All medicines carry some degree of risk, but taking HRT within a few years of your menopause generally has more benefits than risks. As already mentioned, there is a risk of endometrial cancer if insufficient progestogen is given to women who have a uterus. There is a small risk of DVT or PE. This risk is around 1.7 per 1000 women over 50 and is greatest in the first year after you start taking HRT. This risk can be avoided if HRT is given through the skin.

In terms of cardiovascular disease, the biggest risk seems to be for women over 60 who start taking HRT for the first time or women who already have coronary heart disease (CHD). In these situations, there is a possible increased risk of CHD if using combined HRT and of a stroke if using oral HRT.

Breast cancer risk is probably the one that most women fear. Thankfully the risks are not as substantial as was previously thought. It might be increased a little if you use a combined HRT for over five years over the age of 50. Below 50 you don't need to worry about this. But even so, the risk is small with an extra three or four cases per 1000 women for combined HRT and it's lower still for oestrogen only. Combined HRT with a micronised progesterone is thought to have a lower risk of breast cancer than a synthetic progestogen.

> ### GOOD TO KNOW
>
> Drinking two or more units of alcohol per day or being obese in your post-menopause both result in a higher risk of breast cancer than taking five years of combined HRT. It's important to acknowledge lifestyle factors that increase risk and not just focus on the small potential risk from using HRT.

What if HRT isn't working?

As a general rule, you don't need blood tests to check that your HRT is working because you will know. Remember, the main reason to use it is for symptom control. Blood tests will only give you a snapshot, so how you're feeling is your most important guide. If your symptoms aren't controlled, your dose can be increased or the preparation of HRT changed. You should notice a difference within a couple of months of any change, but it could be much quicker.

Doctors follow guidelines which indicate which doses of what types of HRT they should prescribe. Some menopause specialists prescribe outside these guidelines. If you're offered high doses, it's really important to understand what the potential risks might be and to make an informed choice about whether to take it. There seem to be differences in how women absorb HRT through the skin which can impact its effectiveness and a blood test might be needed to check.

It's also important to consider whether your symptoms are actually due to menopause at all or whether they're the result of another condition. It's very easy to think you just need more and more hormones when that isn't indicated.

WHAT ABOUT TESTOSTERONE?

As it stands in the UK, testosterone is only licensed for women who are already on a full dose of oestrogen (and progestogen if they have a uterus) and have low libido. It's frequently used off licence or outside the prescribing guidelines for a number of other reasons and there are many women who say it is the missing part of the jigsaw puzzle for them.

The problem is that we don't know for sure what the long-term consequences of giving a woman testosterone are. Unlike oestrogen and progesterone, blood levels need to be checked to make sure they stay within a recommended range, but what that safe range should be for women as part of HRT isn't really known and some tests are not as accurate as others. Side-effects of testosterone include hair growth and acne, and many women stop it for those reasons or because it doesn't work for them. It's tricky because we know that testosterone is a female hormone, which our body makes and needs. It helps in a number of body systems, including maintaining bone and muscle strength, mood and sex drive. It seems logical that as levels decline with age and we're symptomatic from those lower levels, then topping them up would help.

As a runner, a bit of testosterone to help with motivation, competitiveness, and muscle strength and power would seem like a good idea. But there just isn't the science to back up using it for these reasons. For those in competitive sport, you need to know that testosterone use is also prohibited by the World Anti-Doping Agency (WADA) as it is performance enhancing.

We definitely need more research here. There's not enough evidence to support the prescribing of testosterone as a routine part of HRT at the moment. Some women find it helpful, others don't. If you feel you need it or are offered it, then discuss the pros and cons with your doctor. You need to give informed consent, so it's essential that you have all your questions answered and feel confident that using testosterone outside its licence is the right thing for you.

> 'Menopause has affected me in many different ways, many of them negatively, but using HRT, including testosterone, was a game-changer for me.'
> **Susan Reynolds,** Harrogate

HOW WILL HRT AFFECT MY RUNNING?

HRT can have both positive and negative effects on your running. For some women, taking HRT is the difference between them running or not running. If you're sleeping better, feel more motivated and have fewer joint pains, then that can make you able to run. In this situation it's important to remember that the benefits HRT is giving you also extend to the benefits that being able to be physically active give you, too. This is often overlooked. Here are some of the running-related benefits of HRT:

- Better sleep giving you more energy to run and improved recovery afterwards.
- Fewer joint and muscle aches and pains, making running feel more comfortable.
- Better body temperature control.
- Increased motivation and drive to stick to your runs.
- A less irritable bladder.

Of course, there may be some side-effects of HRT that make running difficult. Here are some that can potentially have an impact on your running:

- **Vaginal bleeding**: This can be irregular at first. You might have stopped your periods but go back to regular bleeds with a cyclical HRT.
- **Breast tenderness**: Both oestrogen and progestogens can cause breast discomfort which makes running uncomfortable.

- **Bloating and fluid retention**: These can make you feel 'heavy' when you run.
- **Muscle cramps**: You might think the cramp is just from the running, but HRT might be contributing.
- **Headaches**: Some women find HRT makes their headaches better, for others it's a trigger. See your doctor if they're persisting beyond a week or are severe.
- **Nausea**: This usually wears off as you get used to the hormones. It's more common if you're taking a hormone in tablet form; in which case try taking it with food.
- **Diarrhoea**: Not what a runner needs but usually settles down within a week or so.
- **Tiredness**: Progesterone can make some women feel drowsy; if so, then taking it at night can help.

Side-effects usually settle down within the first three to six months. Speak to your doctor if they don't.

Weight gain is not a proven side-effect of HRT. In fact, some women find that they lose weight (see chapter 12).

HRT PATCHES, GELS AND EXERCISE

Using skin patches is a great way to take HRT, but runners sweat and shower a lot and some women find their patches come off and they have to change them early. Patches should be put below the waist. On your buttocks or thighs is ideal, but this can mean they're in a prime location for friction from your running kit. When you pull your knickers and running leggings up and down, it can catch on the edge of the patch. Try putting them somewhere this is less likely to happen and away from any elastic.

To get maximum stick, make sure your skin is really clean and dry when you put a patch on. If your skin has any moisturiser or anti-chafing lubricant on it, the patch won't stick well. Using an alcohol-based wipe can help to get the skin really clean, but dry it thoroughly afterwards. When you put the patch on, place your fingers over it and apply gentle pressure for 10 seconds to get a good seal. You could then try using a warm hairdryer over the patch for 10 seconds to get the adhesive warmed up and pressing on the patch for a second time. If it keeps coming off, you can try using a transparent medical dressing such as Tegaderm™ over the top. If this still doesn't work, ask for a different brand or switch to a gel or spray instead.

If you're using an oestrogen gel, you shouldn't have a shower for a few hours afterwards. If you're a morning runner, wait until you've done your run, had your shower and then apply the gel. Otherwise you'll just be washing it off before it's had a chance to be fully absorbed.

GOOD TO KNOW

It's important to remember that HRT is not a contraceptive, because the hormone levels are too low. You need to continue contraception until two years after your last period if you are under 50 and one year if you are over 50. All women can generally stop contraception at age 55.

USING CONTRACEPTIVES FOR HRT

The combined oral contraceptive pill (COCP) contains much higher doses of oestrogen and progestogen than HRT and it can be used to treat menopause symptoms in some women. The risks of taking the COCP increase with age, but if you are fit and healthy, don't smoke and aren't overweight it could be an option for you in early perimenopause if you need contraception, too. The risks would tend to outweigh the benefits after 50. You can't use the COCP alongside HRT.

The progestogen-only pill (POP), on the other hand, can be used alongside HRT and you can continue it for as long as you need contraception. It can't be used as the main progestogen element of combined HRT. If you are using an IUS for contraception, then provided it is the correct type and is less than five years old, it can be used for the progestogen element of HRT. An IUS is a favourite choice for runners, because it tends to stop periods in the majority of women (see chapter 6). An IUS gives you great contraception, and if and when you want HRT you can just rub, spray or stick on a bit of oestrogen. It's not known yet whether the contraceptive implant or injection, which are both progestogen-only contraceptives, can be used for the progestogen part of HRT. They may not offer good enough endometrial protection and aren't licensed to be used in this way.

VAGINAL OESTROGEN

Using vaginal oestrogen is an easy, safe and effective way of reducing menopause symptoms affecting your vulva, vagina and bladder. When oestrogen levels fall, these tissues quite quickly become dry, less elastic and easily irritated. This can lead to a host of symptoms, including painful sex, urinary frequency and vaginal itch (see chapter 8).

Vaginal oestrogen comes as a cream, gel or pessary (tablet) which you insert into your vagina using an applicator. There are also vaginal rings which slowly release oestrogen. Giving oestrogen vaginally results in the bulk of the oestrogen working locally on the nearby tissues and only minimal amounts going into the bloodstream. This amount is so small that you don't need to use a progestogen alongside vaginal oestrogen and it's why it's largely safe for most women. Vaginal oestrogen is now available over the counter. You usually start with a two-week course of daily use and then drop to a maintenance dose of twice a week, with most women experiencing benefit within a couple of months. It's generally easiest to use before you go to bed so most is absorbed by the time you get up. You might want to pop a panty liner in your undies if you're running soon after using vaginal oestrogen as inevitably some will dribble out.

NON-HRT TREATMENTS

There are options if you can't or don't want to use HRT. Most of these are helpful in reducing vasomotor symptoms (flushes and sweats) and mental health symptoms such as depression or anxiety. These treatments can also be used alongside HRT. Each has their own benefits and dosing instructions, cautions and contraindications which are beyond the scope of this book. Some of the treatments are mentioned more specifically in the relevant chapters. Use this list as the basis for your own research and as a prompt for discussion with your doctor.

Cognitive behavioural therapy (CBT)

Suggesting a talking therapy does not mean that your menopause symptoms are in your mind. We are yet to understand the full power of controlling our thoughts. Scientific studies have shown that a course of CBT which changes the way you think and act can reduce hot flushes in some women. It can also reduce symptoms of anxiety and depression. CBT-I has been specifically developed to help with insomnia, even if that lack of sleep is due to night sweats (see chapter 4).

Clonidine

Designed and used to lower blood pressure, clonidine can also reduce hot flushes and sweats in some women and is now licensed for this purpose. The mechanism behind this is not fully understood. It's not suitable if you already have low blood pressure and can make you feel dizzy and light-headed. It should never be stopped suddenly due to potential rebound high blood pressure.

Selective serotonin re-uptake inhibitors (SSRIs) and serotonin-noradrenalin re-uptake inhibitors (SNRIs)

These are both groups of antidepressants. The drug of choice for low mood related to menopause is HRT, but when this can't be used, when it doesn't control symptoms or when depression is not thought to be purely hormone driven, then SSRIs and SNRIs can be tried. As well as benefitting mood, they can ease other menopause symptoms, so may be used specifically for this reason in women when HRT isn't appropriate. For example, paroxetine (SSRI) and venlafaxine (SNRI) may help with hot flushes and sertraline

(SSRI) can reduce anxiety. Make sure you are clear why you are being prescribed a medication, which symptoms are being targeted and what you can expect. It's worth noting that some SSRIs can reduce the effectiveness of tamoxifen which is used to treat breast cancer.

Gabapentin

This is a drug used to treat epilepsy, chronic pain and migraine, but it can reduce hot flushes in around half of the women that use it. It can also help improve sleep. This might be a good choice if sleep and body pain are an issue alongside hot flushes.

Pregabalin

Used to treat epilepsy, anxiety and nerve pain, studies have shown that pregabalin can reduce hot flushes. It may be better tolerated than gabapentin, but is more expensive.

Oxybutinin

This is usually prescribed for overactive bladders, but has been found to reduce hot flushes in some women. It's not licensed for this use, but some specialists might be happy to prescribe it. It can cause a very dry mouth, which limits its use.

Fezolinetant

This new medication licensed for hot flushes is mentioned in chapter 3. It works centrally in the brain to desensitise the body temperature regulation system. It's currently only available on private prescription.

HRT is the gold-standard treatment and none of the above are as effective as HRT, but with patience, trial and error and lifestyle steps, you and your doctor can work towards minimising and controlling your symptoms. As we understand more about menopause and more research is forthcoming, I am hopeful there will be more and better options for those that can't use HRT.

ALTERNATIVE TREATMENTS

There are a range of alternative options that you may find helpful to control your symptoms. This is an area where it's easy to feel confused and overwhelmed, and it's easy to be scammed.

I want to highlight the power of placebo. A placebo is basically a 'dummy drug'. Placebos are often used in clinical trials to test whether the effects of a new drug are real. Half the participants are given the new drug and half are given the placebo, which looks exactly the same but has no active ingredient. Trial participants won't know which one they are taking. Unbelievably, in a study involving people with migraine, the placebo effect was up to 50 per cent as effective as the real drug, even when people knew they were taking a placebo. The very act of taking a treatment has some benefit. This means that despite a placebo not having any effect on the underlying medical condition, you can feel better and have fewer symptoms as a result of taking it. This shows how powerful the brain-body link can be.

The placebo effect must be considered when you think about using an alternative treatment. The effect can be influenced by the branding, price and marketing of the treatment, and how much you believe it will work. It's possible that the treatment you take may help you simply because you use it. That's not necessarily a problem as long as you know that, haven't parted with money you can't afford and are aware those effects may help you initially, but are unlikely to continue in the long term.

Phytoestrogens

These have a similar chemical structure to oestrogens and can be found in certain plants and foods, such as soy, flaxseeds and cruciferous vegetables. Having plenty of these in your daily diet is unlikely to be a bad thing, but whether or not they will definitely have any effect on your menopausal symptoms is unclear.

Isoflavones are a type of phytoestrogen and are found in high levels in soy beans, tofu and red clover. Studies analysing the use of isoflavones for menopause symptoms such as hot flushes haven't shown consistent beneficial results and are largely of poor quality. There are some concerns about consuming large amounts of isoflavones, particularly in terms of breast cancer risk, so they're not recommended for women who have or have had breast cancer. Longer-term studies involving large groups of women are needed to be certain about the safety of using isoflavones and other phytoestrogens in supplements.

Herbal treatments

You will see lots of herbal treatments recommended for controlling menopause symptoms. Here are some of the most commonly used:

- **Black cohosh**: Made from the roots of a plant native to North America, it's not known which chemicals in black cohosh are the active ones when it comes to menopause symptoms or exactly how they work. Studies have shown inconsistent results, with many revealing that black cohosh was no more effective than placebo. There may be some reduction of hot flushes in some women. Again, there is a lack of good quality studies to draw solid conclusions from, particularly looking at the use of black cohosh over more than six months. There's also concern about side-effects, including gastrointestinal upset and significant potential for liver damage. It should be avoided by women using tamoxifen.
- **St John's wort**: Made from a European flowering shrub, this is commonly recommended for menopause symptoms, including vasomotor symptoms, low mood and anxiety. The biggest issue is the potential it has to interact with other medications, including some serious drug interactions with tamoxifen, antidepressants or the contraceptive pill.

- **Evening primrose oil, borage oil and starflower oil**: These all contain gamma-linoleic acid (GLA), an omega-6 fatty acid which may potentially help ease menopausal breast tenderness through its anti-inflammatory effect. It's less likely to help with hot flushes and there really isn't the evidence to back up using it routinely. Some studies show no benefit over placebo and more benefit from lifestyle changes such as exercise.
- **Chinese herbal remedies including ginseng, dong quai and ginko biloba**: Unfortunately, the results from studies looking at Chinese herbal remedies are not positive and found no reduction of hot flushes, anxiety or low mood.

GOOD TO KNOW

Here are the main things you need to know about the difficulty of using herbal treatments safely and effectively:

- These products are not always regulated in the same way that traditional medications are, especially if they are from outside the UK.
- There is inconsistency with unknown quantities of the active ingredient in any one supplement. It may not correlate with what it says on the label and there may be contaminants or even toxic ingredients present.
- There isn't the same level of safety data for alternative treatments.
- Many herbal supplements have the potential to interact with other medications.
- Studies looking at the long-term safety of using these products are often absent.
- Claims of benefit may come from low-quality studies, often performed by the company creating and selling the product.

Should you take them and how do you keep yourself safe if you do? It's important to:

- Do your homework. Read as much as you can and go beyond the marketing page of the seller. Look at quality websites and guidelines such as the British Menopause Society, NICE and menopausematters.co.uk for non-biased opinions.
- Don't just rely on the case-stories you see online. If something sounds too good to be true, it is. Find out who carried out any research studies and whether there are any conflicts of interest.
- Buy from a reputable seller, not a random website or influencer.
- Look for the THR (traditional herbal remedy) stamp on a product. This does not absolutely guarantee its safety but does give some reassurance about the quality and strength of the product.
- If you are taking other medications or have a history of breast or other hormonally linked cancer, speak to your pharmacist or doctor before you start any herbal supplement.
- Be aware of the placebo effect. Monitor your symptoms. If you aren't clear there is any improvement or initial improvement isn't sustained, then stop the supplement. It's easy to find yourself taking something for months and months out of habit when it isn't benefitting you.

Acupuncture

You may find that acupuncture helps to reduce vasomotor symptoms, but the evidence is mixed. It's not clear whether the needling itself causes benefit or the act of spending time with an understanding practitioner. Studies were done with 'sham needles' where needles were used, but not in the locations of known acupuncture points, and the outcomes were the same. Some studies have shown benefits including improving sleep disturbance and easing emotional problems. It's not clear how much is placebo effect, but it's a safe treatment with very few side-effects.

This is not an exhaustive list of menopause treatments but I hope it gives you guidance as to current evidence and helps you to take a critical view of what you try. The key for good menopause treatment is that it suits you as an individual. If a treatment helps your symptoms, isn't causing harm and you are comfortable with the cost and accessibility, then there should be no judgement. We are all different and what works for each of us will vary. Please do remember, though, that a healthy lifestyle surpasses the effectiveness of all these treatments and they should only be used in addition to, not as a replacement for, positive lifestyle steps.

CHAPTER 16

Nutrition

There are entire books written on nutrition in menopause and nutrition for runners, and I don't pretend that a single chapter can replace these. My aim is to give you four simple principles to follow. These are fundamental approaches to your nutrition to keep you from straying into fads and quick fixes, and to ultimately keep you healthy, running and training to the best of your ability through menopause.

I'm very grateful to sports dietician Renee McGregor, from whom I have learned so much, for reviewing this chapter for me and adding her expertise.

1. NOW IS THE TIME

The first principle is simply that now is the perfect time to make a change to what and how you eat, and to adapt your nutrition to the changing demands of your body.

Here are some of the common nutrition complaints and differences that women notice in menopause:

- An increase in hunger.
- Cravings for sweet foods.
- Low energy levels.
- Increased sensitivity to alcohol and caffeine.
- New intolerances of certain foods including running fuels.
- Increased constipation.
- Weight gain and increased body fat.
- Bloating.
- Previous run-fuelling strategies don't seem to work anymore.

Many of these changes have been covered in previous chapters, but they can be unsettling and frustrating. You might never have had to think much about what, how and when you eat in the past. Suddenly your usual routines and habits don't suit you anymore, and you're forced into change. On the other hand, you may be actively seeking change, because of an increasing awareness of the importance of good nutrition for long-term health. Whether forced or intentional, as an active woman this transition in life is the perfect opportunity to take stock, reflect and make some really positive changes to your nutrition, to make you feel better, enjoy life and running more, and have a healthier future.

2. EAT ENOUGH

An easy trap to fall into is not eating enough. Sometimes this is because you're busy or don't appreciate how much you need to eat. Perhaps you have restricted eating due to medical reasons or simply don't have a big appetite. In menopause, however, it's often due to a desire to lose weight. If your waistline is expanding, the immediate reaction is to drop your calorie intake and try to diet it away. This might have worked for you in the past, but in menopause it often has minimal effect. This can lead to further calorie restriction, leaving you feeling miserable, hungry and tired with less motivation to do anything about it. You beat yourself up for not succeeding and you give up. Many women then overeat and end up gaining more weight. This is a dreadful cycle to be in. We need a complete mindset shift in our relationship with food so that we can work with our body and not constantly be resentfully fighting against it.

There are several problems with not eating enough. The first is that feeling hungry isn't a pleasant sensation – it's designed to make us take action and find food. The regulation of hunger hormones is affected by oestrogen levels; ghrelin increases our appetite and leptin suppresses it and it's common to get appetite changes in menopause. Hunger makes people short-tempered, grumpy and unable to concentrate. If you're struggling with the mood changes of menopause, hunger is only going to exacerbate them. Not responding to your body's hunger cues and denying yourself of what you need doesn't foster a good relationship with your body.

Secondly, when you're hungry, the body switches into storage mode, because it doesn't know how many food-free hours are ahead. It stockpiles, storing any energy it does get as fat, which is counterproductive if you're trying to reduce body fat. It also looks for other sources of energy in the body, so starts breaking down muscle, which, again, is not what our menopausal body needs.

Thirdly, not eating enough results in low energy levels, which doesn't help us run and train well, and enjoy our exercise. We need more energy than less active women. It's easy to compare what we eat to what we see others putting on their plates, especially on social media, but each of us has very different lifestyles and different nutritional requirements. It's not just how much we run, it's what we do at work and in our free time. A sedentary office worker will have a lower energy requirement than a busy nurse, even if they're both runners. We need to find what is right for us as individuals.

GOOD TO KNOW

If you're trying to lose weight you do need to be in a calorie deficit, but the key is for it to be a small one and to lose weight very slowly. Around 100 calories deficit per day doesn't sound like much but it's a good goal to aim for to produce sustainable weight loss from body fat. This can easily be achieved by increasing your training a little or making a food switch. Consistency is key and you will lose weight over months and years (around 10 pounds or 4.5 kilograms per year) in a healthy way. This also highlights how a very small increase in our daily calorie intake over a year can lead to weight gain.

Energy deficiency

There are harmful consequences of being constantly energy deficient. In a state of low energy availability (LEA), in an attempt to save energy, the body switches off or down regulates non-essential functions. It has to give you the energy you're using to run, walk and move, and the energy your body needs for basic functions such as breathing and heartbeats, but when there's not enough energy to go around it makes savings in other areas. The impact of energy deficiency can be far reaching and damaging for your body. Hormonal systems which drive normal bodily function become disrupted. Here are some of the ways your body systems can be affected by energy deficiency:

- Reproductive system – irregular or absent ovulation and periods.
- Digestive system – constipation and bloating.
- Musculoskeletal system – muscle cramps and weakness, frequent injury, reduced running performance, bone stress and reduced bone mass.
- Immune system – poor recovery, recurrent infections.
- Brain – disrupted sleep, brain fog, lack of motivation, anxiety, difficulty controlling body temperature.

If you're constantly in energy deficiency and LEA is having an impact on your body, you may have relative energy deficiency in sport (REDs). This is a complex medical condition which can impact any and sometimes multiple body systems. It should be diagnosed and treated by specialists. It can be mild and quickly reversible or severe with the risk of long-term health consequences.

REDs is underpinned by the balance between the energy you take in and the energy you expend. Energy input comes from the calories you consume and energy expenditure is what is used by your normal body function and the activity you do. It's easier than you think to get the balance wrong and slip into energy deficiency. Either not eating enough or training too excessively for the energy you have consumed can result in a negative energy balance. REDs can come from intentionally seeking a large calorie deficit, such as when restricting food or exercising excessively with an eating disorder, but it can also be unintentional. Simply being unaware of the amount of energy you need to consume for your activity level can accidentally result in REDs.

Treatment involves an in-depth assessment of your nutrition, your activity levels and your current state of physical and mental health. Depending on the severity of your condition you may need input from other specialists. It's not as simple as just cutting back on your running and eating a bit more. If you think you may have REDs, seek a referral to an experienced sports dietician.

> ### GOOD TO KNOW
>
> Take another look at the list of ways your body can be affected by energy deficiency. It's easy to see why there is a risk of women being misdiagnosed with perimenopause when in fact they have REDs. For example, if you're an active woman who isn't fuelling adequately for the miles you're running and your periods have become irregular, you aren't running well and have recurrent injuries, you might be perimenopausal or have REDs, or indeed both.

Hopefully I've shown the importance of eating enough and the need to adjust what you eat according to your activity levels and vice versa. I want you to enjoy your food and have plenty of energy to run. Nourishing and fuelling yourself well is preferable to living in a constant state of deprivation. Please make sure you are eating enough.

3. TIME YOUR EATING

The third principle is to carefully consider the timing of your meals and snacks to give you energy at the right time. You don't need a rigid routine that means you can't impulsively go out for dinner with your friends, just some knowledge about what will serve you best.

Eating before a run

Runners need energy and that means available glucose in the bloodstream to fuel muscles. There are studies suggesting that exercising in a fasted state isn't beneficial for menopausal women, especially when it comes to performance. This certainly reflects what women tell me. If you've suddenly found your early-morning runs are harder to do and recover from, adding in a small snack before a run could be a game-changer. It's not just fasted runs first thing in the morning, if you've had a light, early lunch, or skipped lunch altogether and then run after work, you may essentially be running fasted. Those poorly fuelled runs can be hard, unenjoyable and less effective. If you run in the evenings, eating a decent lunch and adding a quick snack before you run is far better.

It's tricky if you're someone who needs to leave a couple of hours between eating and running to allow for digestion. If you're just doing a short run, you don't have to eat a lot – a banana, a handful of raisins or half a bagel with honey will do. You can also use liquids such as a glass of orange juice or some chocolate milk – just something to give you easily available, simple carbohydrate. Try it and see.

Setting yourself up for a good run isn't just about what you eat immediately before. What you've had in the previous 24 to 48 hours makes a difference, too, particularly if you're running long distances. Your body stores carbohydrate in the form of glycogen in your muscles and liver. This can be quickly broken down to glucose and it's important that these stores are full before you run. Eating well the day before your run will top these up and mean you aren't starting out with low glycogen stores. If you have a two-hour run planned for Saturday afternoon, you need to eat well on Friday, not just on Saturday morning.

Eating regularly and well will ensure you have good energy levels throughout the day. Cravings are more likely if you're really hungry. If you frequently forage through the fridge and cupboards looking for quick fixes, then have a look at your meal times and content. When does this normally happen? Can you eat more in the meal before, move the following meal to earlier or plan a healthy snack around that time? Most of us eat the majority of our calories in our evening meal when we might be better served by a bigger breakfast and a main meal at lunchtime. Observe your habits, see when your energy peaks and troughs, and adapt your nutrition to work for you.

> 'I ran fasted in the mornings through my teens, twenties and thirties, but I definitely can't do it anymore, it gives me migraines and nausea.'
>
> **Claire Callaghan**, Bristol

GOOD TO KNOW

Intermittent fasting (IF) is very popular. This is when you choose a restricted window within which you will eat, for example, fasting for 16 hours and eating within an eight-hour slot. It's also called time-restricted eating (TRE). A lot of studies have now been done to look at the effectiveness of this as a tool for weight loss and general health. Ultimately, the findings are that there are no benefits over traditional calorie-controlled diets. However, it's a simple routine that's easy to follow and sustain, and can help some people achieve weight loss and improve body composition. A recent systematic review found that IF could achieve these benefits without losing muscle mass or power. There were negative effects on performance during Ramadan, but these may be influenced by other factors such as hydration. Essentially, IF might be a helpful way to control your calorie intake, but to avoid exercising in a fasted state you might have to adjust your training schedule.

Eating during a run

Glycogen stores only last so long. It varies between individuals, but if you're running at a moderate pace, they'll supply you with carbohydrate for about 90 to 120 minutes. After that time you'll need to top up with simple carbohydrates that you can eat on the go. This is when you might want to use sports fuel such as gels, chews or drinks, which can be more convenient but aren't otherwise superior to natural food stuffs.

Some women in menopause find that their gut becomes more sensitive and they can no longer chug down gel after gel because of nausea, heartburn or diarrhoea. Look for sports fuel made from natural ingredients or switch to normal food such as dates or pieces of white bagel with jam on. Take care with dried fruit as it has a high fibre and fructose content that can upset your gut. Remember that it's really important to keep hydrated while you run. In menopause you can sweat much more than you used to, so your fluid requirement is higher. You might find that you don't feel as thirsty, so you may have to make a conscious effort to drink.

Eating after a run

If you're struggling with energy levels or aren't recovering well, look at what you eat post-run. After a run is when you get fitter, not during the run itself, so you want to provide the optimum environment to gain from your efforts. What you do after a run will also help you with your next one. Taking on some carbohydrate to top up glycogen stores is important. You also need to consume protein for muscle repair and growth, to help you recover and get stronger. A snack with a mix of carbs and protein is therefore ideal. My favourites include chocolate milk and banana, a bagel with peanut butter or a poached egg on toast. I'll have a glass of milk with some almonds or Brazil nuts or a protein shake if I don't feel like eating much.

It's common to lose your appetite after a long run, because the hunger hormone ghrelin can be suppressed. There is some evidence that eating within 30 minutes of finishing your exercise will give you the optimum recovery, but it's not felt to be as important as it was. Try it and see if you feel the benefit. If you struggle to eat after a run, choose a liquid option and return to solid food an hour or so later. Even if you've snacked, have a decent meal within a couple of hours of finishing a run.

If you've sweated excessively or over a long period of time, have a drink containing electrolytes straight after running. You'll get some sodium and potassium in the foods you eat, depending on your choices, but it's convenient to have a big glass of water with an electrolyte tablet dropped into it or make your own by diluting some orange juice and adding a pinch of salt. Eating and rehydrating well can help to stave off post-run headaches too. Hydration and replenishing electrolytes might not be something you've had to consider much before, but it's definitely worth paying attention to if your sweat rate has increased and you're struggling with your running and recovery.

> 'I can't run more than 2 to 3 kilometres without food first. I start to feel light-headed and tremble if I try and go further.'
> **Hilary**

> ### GOOD TO KNOW
> We tend to think of protein as something we need after exercise to help repair muscles. While this is true, it's important to know that it's better to have protein at each snack and meal throughout the day, rather than just a huge protein hit after exercise. Our body is only able to absorb so much at one time. Remember that protein can be an energy source, too, and it's not just carbohydrates that fuel us, so a little in pre-run food and a bigger amount in post-run food is ideal.

4. CHOOSE QUALITY FOODS

Remember there is no 'good' and 'bad' food, there's only food. You don't have to 'earn' food and you shouldn't be running simply to burn off the food you've eaten. If you're slipping into those thoughts, take a step back and consider your relationship with both food and running. Food should be enjoyed and you should run because you want to, not because you feel you have to. It's easy for our relationship with food to deteriorate when we hit perimenopause. If our body changes feel out of control, we may turn to our control of what we eat, which might result in under- or overeating. I encourage you to think differently. Think of food as something that can help you with your running and with your menopause. Rather than focus on what you can take out of your diet, concentrate on what you can add in. This is the perfect time to fill our plate with things that will improve our health. If we're doing this, we have a mindset of abundance rather than scarcity and we're much less likely to eat low-quality, nutrient-poor foods that don't serve us. Let's look at what we should be putting plenty of into our shopping basket at this point in our lives.

Macronutrients

There are three macronutrients (macros) – carbohydrate, protein and fat – and they are all energy sources for the body:

- **Carbohydrate:** The body's primary energy source, particularly when it comes to exercise; this is because carbohydrate is easily broken down into glucose to fuel us. There are two different types of carbohydrate: simple carbohydrates, which are easily digested and get glucose quickly into the bloodstream, and complex carbohydrates, often called starchy carbs, which take longer to digest and provide a longer-lasting level of energy. Simple carbs are great for a quick boost of energy before and during a run, but when it comes to our regular meals we need to focus more on the complex carbs. These will help to even out our energy levels through the day. A portion of starchy, complex carbs will give you a satisfying meal.

Shopping basket: potatoes and sweet potatoes, wholegrain bread, wholegrain pasta, brown rice, oats, couscous, quinoa, wholegrain cereals, bananas.

- **Protein:** This is a big one when it comes to active women, because most of us aren't eating enough. Protein is made of chains of amino acids and has multiple functions in the body, including roles in making hormones and enzymes, transporting and storing nutrients, and building and repairing body tissues such as muscle and bone. It's an energy source too. An adequate protein intake is essential in menopause, because we are losing both bone and muscle mass. If we want to maintain and build these, we need to give our body the building blocks, and protein contains these. I think it's important to get a rough idea of how much protein an active woman needs, because it's more than you might think. A standard recommended amount for an average adult is 0.75 grams per kilogram of bodyweight per day. For a 60-kilogram woman, this would be 45 grams. An endurance runner, however, is recommended to have around 1.4 grams per kilogram, which would be 84 grams if you weigh 60 kilograms. There are some scientists recommending up to 2.4 grams per kilogram for active women in menopause, which is 144 grams through the day for a 60-kilogram woman. An average chicken breast contains around 50 grams of protein, 150 grams of Greek yoghurt will give you 15 grams of protein and an egg will give you 5 grams. It's possible and ideal to consume enough protein through natural food stuffs, but if you're struggling, protein shakes can be convenient. Adding protein to each meal and snack throughout the day is better than one large load. After exercise, aim for around 0.4 grams per kilogram, which would be 24 grams for a 60-kilogram woman.

Shopping basket: chicken and turkey breasts, red meat, tinned tuna, oily fish, seafood, tofu, tempeh, eggs, Greek yoghurt, cottage cheese, cow's milk and soy milk, beans and pulses, nuts, seeds.

- **Fat:** Years of being told to avoid fat has led to many of us being afraid to go near it and choosing low-fat options whenever we can. Low-fat options are often inferior choices as they're usually loaded with sugar to maintain taste. Fat is essential for the normal functioning of our body. It keeps us warm, protects and cushions our organs and helps us absorb fat-soluble vitamins, such as A, D, E and K. It has a role in our immune system, provides essential fatty acids and is a great energy store. These are just some of the clever things fat does in our body, but excess fat intake can lead to obesity, high cholesterol and an increased risk of cardiovascular disease. You should avoid eating large amounts of saturated fats, trans fats and ultra-processed foods. Fat is, however, an important part of a balanced diet and we should be aiming for around 1 gram per kilogram of bodyweight per day. Our best source of fat is from wholefoods and we want to choose foods with a high content of unsaturated fats as they contain essential fatty acids. Polyunsaturated fats can help to lower LDL cholesterol, high levels of which can increase heart disease and stroke risk. Don't exclude fat, but choose your fat wisely.

Shopping basket: nuts and nut butters, seeds, oily fish (salmon, sardines, mackerel), avocados, olive oil, rapeseed oil, sunflower oil, eggs, a small amount of dark chocolate.

Micronutrients

Micronutrients are the vitamins and minerals that our body needs to perform all its functions and keep us healthy. There are too many to mention them all, but the take-home message is that with a balanced, varied and diverse diet, you can get enough of all of them from what you eat, with the exception of vitamin D and, if you're eating a plant-based diet, vitamin B12. There are a few micronutrients that are particularly relevant to menopause:

- **Iron:** Around 8 per cent of women in the UK population have a degree of iron deficiency, largely due to diets which contain insufficient iron. Iron is needed to make red blood cells and women and girls are at particular risk of iron deficiency due to losing blood during periods. In perimenopause, periods can often get more frequent and heavier before they fizzle out and this means a higher risk of iron deficiency. We're also at increased risk because we're runners and endurance sports lead to an increased iron consumption. Iron deficiency can make you feel tired, make your hair fall out and give you a headache, among other symptoms, but it can also lead to iron-deficiency anaemia (see chapter 5). It's easy to add lots of iron-rich foods to your diet.

Shopping basket: red meat, the dark meat on chicken and turkey, eggs, leafy green vegetables, fish and seafood, dried apricots, nuts, seeds, beans and pulses (chickpeas are great), iron-fortified bread and cereals.

GOOD TO KNOW

Vitamin C can increase iron absorption so have a small glass of orange juice or a vegetable which is rich in vitamin C, such as red pepper or broccoli, along with your main meal. Caffeine, on the other hand, can inhibit iron absorption, so is best avoided during and immediately after meals.

- **Vitamin D:** This is the one vitamin supplement we need to take. It's made by our body when direct sunlight hits our skin. Specific vitamin D receptor cells in skin convert cholesterol into vitamin D when they are exposed to ultraviolet B (UVB). Vitamin D is important, because it helps the absorption of calcium from the gut and is critical for bone formation. It also has a role in our immune system and our muscle and brain function. Sunlight is in short supply in many areas of the world and skin needs to be exposed for the receptor cells to be activated. There are foods which are rich in vitamin D and as runners we probably get more sun exposure than most people, but it's still hard to get adequate amounts from diet and sun alone. We also have to balance the risks of sun damage (see chapter 13). Taking a daily supplement of 10 to 25 micrograms during autumn and winter is recommended and you can continue this all year if you live somewhere there is little sun, have darker skin pigment or you cover your skin for religious or preference reasons. We don't know what the maximum safe dose is for individuals so, unless you've been advised to take them by a medical professional, be wary of very high-dose supplements which can be as strong as 1250 micrograms.

Shopping basket: beef, liver, egg yolks, oily fish, cheddar, foods that are fortified with vitamin D such as some cereals, milk and spreads. A vitamin D supplement, no fancy, expensive one is needed, plain vitamin D is fine.

- **Vitamin B12:** With a rising number of women choosing to eat plant-based diets, and a higher risk of being deficient in B12 when you're over 50, it's important to mention vitamin B12 (cobalamin) supplements. B12 is another essential micronutrient which has multiple roles in the body including in the brain and nervous system, red blood cell production and DNA synthesis. A deficiency in B12 might show up as anaemia, fatigue or numbness and tingling in hands and feet. Most foods that contain B12 are animal-based, so if you are vegetarian or vegan it's important to take a daily B12 supplement of 10 micrograms daily.

Shopping basket: red meat, chicken and turkey, fish and shellfish, eggs, milk, cheese, yoghurt, yeast extract (marmite or Vegemite), fortified food such as cereals and plant-based milks, fortified tofu.

- **Calcium:** I mention calcium not because I want you to take a calcium supplement, but instead to tell you that you probably don't need to. Calcium is essential for healthy bones and also for muscle function and blood clotting. A deficiency can lead to an increased risk of bone fracture, but unless you have excluded dairy from your diet, then supplementation isn't usually required. It's easy to get the recommended amount of 700 milligrams from your daily diet. Taking too much calcium can give gastrointestinal side-effects and even be harmful, so it's not a supplement to take routinely unless you have been advised to do so. If you're vegan, it's harder to reach recommended levels but it can be done.

Shopping basket: milk, cheese, yoghurt, green leafy vegetables but not spinach which can reduce calcium absorption, sardine and pilchards (those tiny fish bones are full of calcium), plant-based milks which are fortified with calcium, fortified bread products, soya, nuts, beans.

- **Omega-3 fatty acids:** These are polyunsaturated fatty acids which are important for a healthy heart and brain as well as supporting your immune and hormonal systems. If you eat oily fish twice a week, you'll likely get enough omega-3s. If you don't, then you can add nuts and seeds to your breakfast to give you a good supply. Supplements are no longer routinely recommended, because the evidence for their benefit in preventing conditions such as cardiovascular disease is inconclusive. If you feel you fall short of omega-3s you can consider a supplement, but choose an omega-3 rather than fish liver oil which may contain high levels of vitamin A which can be harmful over the long term.

Shopping basket: oily fish, walnuts, ground flaxseed, pumpkin seeds, chia seeds, rapeseed and linseed oil, soya beans, soya milk and tofu.

- **Magnesium**: There are all sorts of magnesium preparations available that are targeted at women in menopause. You can rub it on your skin, bathe in it and eat it in a variety of forms. Unless you have a magnesium deficiency, there is no need for you to take a supplement; you can get all you need from your daily diet. Having said that, there are many women who say that taking magnesium has helped with their anxiety symptoms or poor sleep. Magnesium is important for healthy bones and muscles, and as an active woman your magnesium requirements are higher than average, partly because magnesium is lost in sweat. If you feel your diet is low in magnesium, then magnesium supplementation is a fairly safe option to try. The recommended daily target for magnesium is 320 milligrams, although this may be higher in active women. Large doses can give you gastrointestinal side-effects and excess doses can be harmful. Magnesium can be absorbed in small amounts through the skin but the evidence points to the oral route being superior.

Shopping basket: nuts (almonds and cashews in particular), seeds, leafy green vegetables, dark chocolate, beans, lentils, wholegrains.

Good to Know

There are lots of tracking apps to assess your nutrition in more detail. They can give you a rough guide as to the quantity and quality of your diet, and can also be a motivational tool to keep you on track if you're trying to make improvements. Do keep in mind that they can be very inaccurate and don't replace seeing a dietician, who can calculate your requirements and intake in an individualised way. It depends on your personality and relationship with food, but it's very easy to fall into obsessive behaviour with tracking apps, so consider carefully whether they are a good option for you. Remember to aim for a balanced and varied diet over a week rather than obsessing over every individual day.

The gut microbiome

A discussion about quality foods and menopause would be incomplete without mention of the gut microbiome (see chapter 9). Focus on feeding your gut bacteria with a diverse range of foods. Choosing fruit and vegetables of different colours is a good place to start – aim to eat a rainbow over the week. These, along with wholegrain foods, are fibrous foods that contain prebiotics which feed your gut bacteria and help them to grow. Probiotics, on the other hand, actually contain bacteria which contribute to the microbiome. You'll find these in fermented foods and they're preferable to taking probiotic supplements.

Shopping basket: a wide variety of different vegetables and fruit, legumes, wholegrain foods, healthy fats, fermented foods such as kombucha, kefir, kimchi, yoghurt with live cultures, sauerkraut and tempeh.

Fibre

Fibre is not a food group on its own; it's a hard-to-digest carbohydrate found in plants and there are both soluble and insoluble types of fibre. It's really important to eat enough of it because a high-fibre diet will:

- Prevent constipation.
- Feed your gut microbes.
- Lower harmful cholesterol levels (soluble fibre).
- Lower your risk of cardiovascular disease, including heart disease and stroke.
- Lower your risk of type 2 diabetes.
- Help control blood glucose levels.
- Reduce your risk of bowel cancer and possibly breast cancer.
- Help you to feel full after you've eaten.
- Help maintain a healthy weight.

Aim for around 30 grams of fibre each day. Most of us don't manage that, but hitting your 'five a day' fruit and vegetable target will help, and so will swapping to wholegrain versions of white foods. Avoid too much fibre right before a run as it's hard to digest, so opt for a low-fibre snack. If you have digestive issues, such as irritable bowel syndrome (IBS), you may have to find a careful balance of fibre that works for you.

Shopping basket: soluble fibre – oats, quinoa, apples, oranges, bananas, dried fruit, beans, lentils, peas, carrots, brussel sprouts, kale, sweet potato, onions, leeks. Insoluble fibre: wholegrain bread, wholewheat pasta, brown rice, bran, potatoes, green beans, cauliflower, nuts.

Collagen and creatine

Both collagen and creatine are plastered all over social media and large numbers of women I know are taking one or the other or even both. However, remember the overarching fact that you can get all the nutrition you need from a healthy, balanced diet.

Collagen is a protein found in our skin, muscles, tendons, connective tissue and bones. It has other roles in the body, but it's largely a structural protein. A diet rich in protein from animal and marine sources supplies our body with collagen, particularly if we eat the skin of meat and fish or cook meat with the bones in. Gelatin is also very rich in collagen. As we get older, the amount of collagen in our body reduces because our production of it slows down and it gets broken down more quickly. This loss speeds up around menopause and results in a change in our skin, hair and musculoskeletal tissues.

Despite what you might see online, the evidence for using collagen supplements to slow down the ageing process isn't conclusive. In fact, the more robust studies point to it not having any effect. Supplements may potentially help skin, with one systematic review and meta-analysis finding a reduction in wrinkles and improved elasticity and hydration of skin after 90 days of taking hydrolysed collagen. Note that skin creams containing collagen have no effect as collagen molecules are too big to pass into the skin. For hair and nails, the evidence is mixed and much is of low quality but there seems to be little benefit. In terms of bones, joints and muscles, there really isn't enough evidence yet to suggest we all need to take collagen but there may be some benefits, particularly in post-menopause. Collagen is generally safe to take, so if you can't increase the collagen in your diet and you want to use a supplement, then go ahead. Read Renee's note on collagen on the next page.

Creatine is something you might want to consider taking if you are looking for maximum gains in athletic performance and muscle-building. It's made from three amino acids and it's found in our muscles and brain. We can get it from meat, fish and eggs, but it isn't present in plant-based foods. Our body also makes its own from the protein we eat. Around 95 per cent of the body's creatine is stored in muscles and it's used to produce energy, particularly during short, high-intensity moves such as sprinting or lifting weights. It's unlikely to be useful for building our running endurance.

It's not known how each individual person will respond to creatine in terms of the gains they make. There's a range of potential side-effects, including stomach upsets and dizziness, and care needs to be taken in people who are at risk of or have existing kidney disease. Creatine pulls water into muscles and it's essential to be well hydrated if you use it. At the moment, its best use seems to be taking it daily alongside regular resistance training to improve muscle growth and strength. There's doubt over its benefit on bone strength, and its impact on wider health issues such as depression, cognitive levels and heart health are still being researched. We don't know what the effects of taking creatine for more than a few years are.

Meet the expert: Renee McGregor

Renee McGregor is a leading sports dietician with over 25 years of experience working in clinical and performance nutrition. She has managed sport science teams leading into the Rio 2016 Olympics and provided team management on numerous occasions at major championships in a variety of sports. She is one of the UK's leading voices in athlete health, the female athlete, REDs and hormonal health, and works with a number of teams and brands on a consultancy basis, providing expert support on REDs, and ensuring nutritional and clinical guidance for both performance and health.

Renee is a best-selling author whose latest book *Fuel for Thought* was an instant success. She writes a monthly column for Runner's World and provides technical support on documentaries, news and media such as for the BBC documentary *Freddie Flintoff: Living with Bulimia* where she was the clinical advisor. Renee is actively involved in trying to improve diversity and equality in both trail and fell running.

When not inspiring others with her incredible work, Renee can be found running the mountains and chasing the trails around her home in the Lake District.

Website: reneemcgregor.com, Instagram: @r_mcgregor

A NOTE FROM RENEE

We are living in an era where nutrition, fitness and our bodies are all controversial subjects. Everyone has an opinion and many are trying to sell you a promise, where they gain financially but you are left with false gold. Whether it's celebrities promoting a particular brand of supplement or an organisation boasting that their nutrition approach is bespoke to your needs, generally someone profits at your expense.

Let's take collagen as an example. There are definitely some benefits to taking collagen for women going through this stage of life. However, not all collagen supplements are equal. Firstly, it's important to know that only bovine collagen has the right type that is going to have any benefits to your connective tissue, bone and joint health, but secondly the dose is really key. Instead I see well-known celebrities promoting brands that are plant-based, which have absolutely no impact on our health and yet will burn a hole in your pocket. Who has benefited? The supplement company and the celebrity, but not you. It's not your fault though, you get sucked in because these celebrities are fundamentally selling you a lifestyle, not a supplement, and frankly are unlikely to have done any research or understanding about whether the product has any benefits or not.

So my final words to you are that when it comes to nutrition, firstly, if it seems too good to be true, it probably is and, secondly, remember to do your research and ask yourself is this trend, approach or message actually relevant to me, my needs, my lifestyle and where I am in this present moment of life?

Let's finish by recapping the four main principles:

1. Now is the perfect time to make a change. You have so much to gain for your health and your running.
2. Make sure you are eating enough. If you are trying to lose weight do it very slowly with a small calorie deficit.
3. Time your eating to benefit your running. Don't run on empty.
4. Choose good quality and diverse foods. Be mindful about what you are eating and do the best you can, most of the time.

CHAPTER 17

Training

Whether your training is going really well or you're struggling to run at all, there are things you need to pay attention to now menopause has hit; adaptations to your training which will benefit your running both now and in the future. We often lose our running confidence in menopause, but if we train in the right way, with the right mindset, it can help us slowly build back confidence and our running will spiral upwards instead of downwards. We often unintentionally set ourselves up to fail. Read on to see how you can set yourself up to succeed instead.

TRAINING ESSENTIALS

I'll cover seven training essentials, then move on to the other elements that make up a good training schedule, but I'm very conscious that getting out for a run at all is sometimes a momentous challenge. The key to running and training in menopause is acknowledging how you feel on any given day and doing what feels right for you at that moment. Something is always better than nothing, even if it's just a short walk. Please know that I see you if this feels impossible at the moment.

1. Meet yourself where you're at

I need you to be really honest with where you are with your running. Not where you were two years ago or think you could be on a really good day with the wind in the right direction and super shoes on your feet. It's in our nature to compare ourselves, to others and to our previous running. Stop looking back through your old stats and pining to be there again. You are not in the same body. Things have changed. It doesn't mean you can't get back to that level, you just have to go about things in a different way. Menopause exposes our weaknesses, and now is the time to strip things back and build from the foundations again.

It might make your toes curl, but you need an honest assessment of your current baseline. Choose an average day and a familiar route. Record your average pace, time or just give yourself a mark out of 10 for how it felt. Don't overthink it, it's just a number, not a reflection of your worth. Also make a note of the number of days a week you run, strength train or cross train. You need to know where you're starting from to be able to show progress and keep yourself motivated. We often feel disappointed with how we're running now compared to how we used to run, but in reality it was a different time in life. You are not a weaker person, you are in menopause, negotiating vast hormonal shifts. You are also older and we need to recognise that not all our issues are due to menopause; some are simply from ageing. You are where you are and that is absolutely fine. Let's build from there.

2. Warm up

Runners just want to run and the first mile is often the warm-up. This needs to change now. Introducing a short warm-up will benefit your run and reduce your injury risk. Your body needs this more as you get older so start now and get a short routine embedded. Here are the areas you need to warm up:

- **Joints**: Synovial fluid lubricates, cushions and nourishes our joints. Movement stimulates its production and circulation. Dynamic stretches and mobilisation pre-run will help protect your joints.
- **Nerves**: The pathways from your brain to your muscles and vice versa are crucial for balance, coordination and injury prevention. Wake them up with exercises standing on one leg, sideways skips and fast footwork.
- **Muscles**: A cold muscle is more likely to be injured than a warm one and a muscle that's been primed during a warm-up will perform better during the run. Resistance bands are perfect for activating key running muscles such as glutes.

- **Cardiovascular system**: During running, we need four to five times as much blood to supply extra oxygen to our muscles and remove the waste products of exercise. To achieve this, our heart pumps faster and more forcefully and our blood vessels dilate. Our body has to fire up its systems, pass chemical messages around the body and adjust to the new demands. Brisk walking and slow jogging will kick-start this process.
- **Lungs**: When running, the rate and depth of your breathing increases to inhale extra oxygen and exhale the waste gas, carbon dioxide. At rest we take around 15 breaths per minute, but that increases to 40 to 60 during running. A brisk walk or jog helps your lungs to prepare for the task ahead.
- **Mind**: Think about what would make a good run for you. Set a realistic aim. It doesn't need to be a distance or time goal; you can decide it's a chilled run to enjoy the scenery. Be clear what you expect of yourself and that this is appropriate for the day you are in. Talk to yourself positively and imagine yourself reaching your target.

You can incorporate all of this in five to 10 minutes. Warm up before you go out the door if you feel self-conscious, or just be proud and set a good example for anyone who cares to watch you. Here's a short warm-up routine that will cover all of the main areas:

1. Foot/ankle circles – 4 times clockwise and anticlockwise on each foot.
2. Hip circles – big wide circles, 4 clockwise and 4 anticlockwise.
3. Torso twist – turn your upper body to look behind you to your right and left 4 times while keeping your hips pointing forwards.
4. Arm swings – big circles, 4 forwards and 4 backwards.
5. Leg swings – use a wall to balance and swing your straight leg forwards and backwards 4 times, then side to side 4 times. Repeat on the other leg.
6. Squats – 8 with or without a resistance band just above your knees.
7. Sideways skip – 4 gallops in each direction 4 times.
8. Fast feet – small, fast steps on the spot, moving forwards, backwards and sideways and/or in a figure of eight pattern.
9. A brisk walk graduating to a slow jog while you set your intention for the run ahead.

> ## GOOD TO KNOW
> There are lots of factors that should influence the length and content of your warm-up. It needs to be longer on cold days or if you're returning from injury or illness. If you have arthritis or musculoskeletal syndrome of menopause, you should spend more time warming up your joints and muscles. If you have ongoing medical conditions such as asthma, then a longer and more gradual heart and lungs warm-up is beneficial. If you're on uneven trails, spend more time focusing on balance and coordination. If it's a sprint session, you need a longer warm-up and lots of emphasis on glutes, quads and arms. Be clever, focused and time efficient. Some kind of warm-up is better than none in menopause and beyond.

3. Run more slowly

Do you have any truly easy runs, where you can chat, feel completely comfortable and as if you could run forever? You might think you do, but you probably aren't going slowly enough. It's so easy to start slowly and find your pace picks up as you go. A very slow run is not a waste of time, it's a powerful tool, especially now you're menopausal. This type of training (often called zone 2 training where your heart rate remains around 60 to 70 per cent of your maximum heart rate), helps to build your aerobic capacity which is how efficiently your muscles can use oxygen and keep going without you feeling tired. It increases the number and size of the energy-producing mitochondria in your muscles and trains those slow-twitch muscle fibres that we have more of than men.

We tend to think only hard runs increase our fitness and discount the benefits of slow running. By introducing easy runs, you will build your aerobic base and this will set you up to run longer distances more easily. The increased mitochondria will benefit your faster runs, too. It's a pace that is much easier to recover from which is vital in menopause when recovery can be slower. If you want to improve any aspect of your running, you need a good amount of slow, very easy, conversational running. A rough guide is that 80 per cent of your runs should feel easy. It takes practice to run more slowly than you usually would, but, honestly, you really need to slow down! This is also reassuring if you've found you've got slower in menopause. Don't be frustrated by this, use it. Perhaps it's our body's way of telling us what it needs. Embrace the slow.

4. Run really fast

I've just told you to slow down and now I'm telling you to speed up, but hear me out! Once you've started building that aerobic base, all I'm asking you to do is take one 20-minute run each week and turn it into something really powerful that will benefit you in many ways. A weekly sprint session will:

- Improve your speed, whether you're slowing down or running well and want to improve your personal bests.
- Build muscle and preserve your fast-twitch muscle fibres, which are the first to go when muscle mass is lost.
- Increase the number and power of energy-producing mitochondria in your muscles.
- Help generate and maintain a healthy body composition by improving visceral-fat burning.
- Improve your blood sugar control.
- Make you feel liberated and powerful.

Sprint interval training (SIT) is not complicated and can be fun. Warm up really well and do a good 10- or 15-minute run before you begin. Find a flat, person- and dog-free, 60m stretch of ground with no trip hazards. You can do this on grass, tarmac or an athletics track. Run as fast as you can along that distance. Try to sustain a 9 out of 10 effort. You should be gasping for breath at the end. Walk or jog around until you get your breath back, which might take two or three minutes. Then do it again. Aim for five sprints initially and as you get more confident and fitter, increase up to eight. Have a good cool-down jog or walk afterwards. An alternative would be 30-second sprints on a static bike with rest periods of easy cycling in between. You'll need to step out of your comfort zone to do this. Don't be afraid, give it a go. You will grow in confidence. I like to do this session with headphones on and power tunes filling my ears. Channelling my inner Olympic sprinter feels great.

> ## GOOD TO KNOW
> VO2 max is a measure of how much oxygen your body can transport and use. Muscles demand a high amount of oxygen during running. VO2 max varies with sex, age and fitness, but your maximum is largely determined by your genetics. VO2 falls with age, but menopause may have some effect, too, so you may see yours reducing. Changes in body composition may account for this with falling muscle mass reducing how much oxygen can be used and a lower maximum heart rate affecting how quickly it can be transported. A small study showed that VO2 max was more affected in women who had a surgical menopause compared to those who had a natural one. Interval training and hill repeats can help to improve your VO2 max. Remember the VO2 max on your sports watch won't be very accurate, but you can observe the trend of your value.

> 'I think getting faster takes longer in menopause.'
> **Jodi Clouston-Kerr**

5. Strength train

Adding strength work to your training is a non-negotiable now you are in menopause. The future you is willing you to read chapter 17 and take action. Don't miss it!

6. Jump and hop

Because you spend time in the air with both feet off the ground, running is essentially jumping. In order to be able to jump we need power and the explosive contraction of muscles to push us off the ground. We're losing that power as our muscle mass declines, but we can retain some of it through explosive movements called plyometrics.

Plyometrics include jumps and hops where you leap off the ground as muscles contract and then those same muscles get stretched as you land. In physics, power is force multiplied by velocity (speed in a certain direction), therefore to gain muscle power we need to jump quickly and with force. Plyometric movements train this. Plyometrics involves multi-direction jumps, which are great for increasing bone strength, although you need to be reasonably strong and stable before you introduce plyometrics, as they're complex movements and to do them effectively you need good coordination and muscle strength.

Plyometrics are hard work for muscles so introduce them gradually and only do them once or twice a week. You can do specific plyometrics sessions or sprinkle them in among your other training. There is quite a high risk of injury with plyometrics, especially when you first start, so don't do them when you're tired (mentally or physically) or when your muscles are fatigued. Concentrate on fewer movements with good form and lots of power. They're great for training your coordination and balance, too.

7. Rest and recover

Rest and recovery is a training essential, especially in menopause. Insufficient recovery can leave you feeling exhausted, not getting the maximum benefits from your running and even ill or injured. It catches up with you at some point. Remember that menopause exposes your weaknesses.

Rest allows your body to adapt to the load you're putting on it. It needs time to repair and strengthen itself before applying more load. Inadequate rest and recovery is a common error in menopause. We can be so set in what has worked for us in the past that we don't acknowledge we need change, or we take rest but with a sense of guilt that we should be exercising more. However, less is often more and remember that sleep is crucial for recovery (see chapter 4).

Plan and take at least two rest days in your normal week of exercising, or more if you feel you need them or you're returning to exercise after a break. You also need 'step back' weeks. Whether you're strength training or following a running training plan, at least every fourth week should be an easier one. This tactic means that you can train sustainably. It might feel like three steps forward and one step back, but you will end up further ahead, in a healthy and strong way. Any training plan you follow should be long enough to account for these step-back weeks and that means training plans for women in menopause should be longer than standard ones, which are generally created around the needs and science of men's bodies. You can also extend your plan by another one or two weeks with emergency 'menopause weeks' that allow you to take a week off or a big step back in order to cope with menopause symptoms.

Recovery also means doing what you feel suits your body and helps you regenerate more quickly. There are a host of alternatives available, from ice baths to foam rolling, compression socks to massage. The evidence for most of these is limited and doesn't specifically include women in menopause, but if you feel something helps you and you're happy with it, then crack on.

GOOD TO KNOW

If you track your heart rate variability (HRV), you are likely to see it reduce in peri- and post-menopause. HRV is a measure of the variation in the time between heartbeats and is a good marker of well-being. A high HRV suggests the heart is able to adjust and adapt to any stressors. A low HRV has been linked to cardiovascular disease, depression and anxiety. Lots of factors affect HRV, including body composition, stress levels, and oestrogen and progesterone levels. There is a lot we don't yet know, but a healthy lifestyle can potentially improve our HRV. Rather than specific values, look for trends over time.

> 'It takes longer to recover now I'm menopausal, so I consciously make sure I have rest days or do some other form of exercise on non-running days.'
>
> **Helen L,** Lancaster

Those are the seven elements to introduce into your running week. Cut right back on those runs where you're always a bit too out of breath to have a chat (zone 4). These make up the bulk of most women's training and there is a place for them, but not for every run you do.

You don't have to make all these changes at once. Small manageable steps are always best. Know your starting point, add in a warm-up and run your easy runs really slowly. Then add in some strength work, sprint-interval training and, when you're ready, some plyometrics. This will give you a really good foundation and help to adapt your training to the changes that are happening in your body. Whether you're aiming to just continue enjoying social running, wanting to crack out a PB or running your first marathon, these are constants you can't do without now. As I keep saying, you might have got away without them so far, but now is the time for change.

GOOD TO KNOW

Please remember that however well you schedule your training, none of it is going to be beneficial if you don't eat properly. Good nutrition and good running go hand in hand. For more about how to nourish yourself well for running, see chapter 16.

> 'The aching, heavy runs were a real shock at first. I was exhausted at 2 miles. I've learned there's nothing you can do except add more rest in between runs and, if going up a kerb feels like a hill, then slow down and make it a shorter run. Also be careful of the other workouts you're doing in the week.'
>
> **Anonymous**

OTHER TRAINING ADAPTATIONS

Aside from these training essentials, there are other things we need to consider when it comes to our menopausal body. Let's look at flexibility and stretching, balance and coordination before moving on to cross training.

Flexibility

Are your toes getting further away? Being less flexible is generally accepted as a natural part of ageing. With the hormonal changes of menopause, tendons and ligaments become stiffer, muscles lose some of their elasticity and soft tissues dry out a bit, which all reduce our flexibility.

What flexibility do you actually need in your day-to-day life? While you might like to take on a 'do the splits in 30 days' challenge, do you really need to be able to do the splits? We all need to be able to reach down and tie up our running shoes or trim our toenails, reach up to high cupboards, do up our own sports bra and climb over a stile. But those of us who aren't professional gymnasts don't need to aim for high degrees of flexibility. In fact, being too flexible isn't helpful for running. We just need to feel comfortable, relaxed in our joints, and able to do the things we need and want to do.

To maintain flexibility, we need to work at it. The reason it reduces as we get older is in large part down to the fact that we do less activity that needs us to be flexible. Some people are naturally more flexible than others and constantly trying to be what you aren't isn't good for your motivation or confidence.

Static stretching

A static stretch is where you hold a muscle in a pose. Doing these before a run may impair performance and won't reduce injury risk. Doing them immediately after a run impedes recovery, because it restricts blood flow in a muscle which needs as much flow as possible through it to bring oxygen and healing cells, and remove waste products. Yes, I'm telling you it's okay to miss your post-run stretch! It's better to stretch half an hour later, after your shower, or to stretch at a different time altogether, after a warm-up of course. It's often the psychological benefits of a relaxed and calm stretching session that do more good than any direct effect on the muscles.

Focus on what you need to stretch. If you feel you're losing a particular movement, then follow a stretching programme and see yourself improve. By all means stretch if it feels good, but my advice is not to become too focused on extreme stretching which doesn't serve any good purpose.

> ### GOOD TO KNOW
>
> The ideal time to hold a stretch is for 15 seconds. Any less and it's unlikely to be beneficial. If you're very flexible or have high goals, then you may need to hold for longer than that, but no more than 45 seconds. Remember that overstretching can lead to injury.

Dynamic stretches

Dynamic stretches take a joint through its complete range of movement. These are ideal to do as part of your warm-up. Done before a run they will help protect joints, wake up the muscles and nerves, and reduce injury risk. They're also a great option for opportunistic exercise, when you're waiting for the kettle to boil or for breaking up your sedentary time. Here are some great dynamic stretches you can do:

- Squats
- Lunges
- Hip circles
- Leg swings
- Arm swings
- Glute bridges
- High knees
- Torso twist
- Jumping jacks.

You don't have to do the whole lot at once. In fact, if you overdo it before a run you'll tire yourself out. Choose a few that feel good and are relevant to your workout.

BALANCE AND COORDINATION

Nerve cells located in muscles, tendons and joints send feedback information to the brain. They inform it of position and movement. This is called proprioception. The brain then responds with instructions about what to do next. This process is vital for us to be coordinated, balanced and accurate in our movements. Firing up these nerve pathways and waking up these lines of communication gets us ready for action, particularly in terms of making sure our joint position sense is activated and our leg joints are stable. This is really important for running, but also for us to be able to do strength work, plyometrics and dynamic stretches effectively and safely.

As we get older, the speed at which these nerve pathways work slows down and if they are unused they can wither away. Lots of women in menopause find they struggle with poor balance and clumsiness, tripping and knocking into things. It's therefore really important that we make a conscious effort to work on and maintain our balance and coordination. Hard work now will reap huge rewards in the future. Going down stairs, negotiating icy pavements and moving out of the way of hazards are all things that some older people find hard to do and can result in falls. Confidence for these everyday activities comes from having strong muscles, and great balance and coordination.

It's simple to train your balance and coordination. From this day forwards, when you're waiting in a queue, standing at your desk or on the phone, introduce some time on one leg. Never brush your teeth standing on two feet. You'll probably notice you are much better on one side and that's normal, but it shows where your weaknesses are and where you need to focus your efforts. Walk toe-heel along the cracks in the pavement, balance on the kerb or on a fallen log. Basically I'm asking you to be a child again.

Mixing up the pace you're doing things and changing direction or rhythm all help to build balance and coordination. You can work on this yourself with skipping, using an agility ladder or playing with the dog. Dance classes and yoga also do wonders for your balance and sense of body position. You will build your balance and coordination through running, especially off-road, through dynamic stretches, plyometrics and strength work, but to be honest you really need a basic level of balance and coordination to do those things well and safely, so invest some time in specific exercises. Your future you is shouting her thanks for every minute you spend working on this. For a strength and balance workout, see chapter 19.

CROSS TRAINING

Cross training is essentially any other exercise you do alongside your running. Examples are cycling (outdoors or on a static bike), swimming or rowing. The elliptical or stair stepper at the gym and hiking count, too. We should all open our minds to the benefits of cross training in menopause. Running is a very repetitive movement using set groups of muscles. To be fit and healthy individuals, and have good body movement and awareness, we'd do well to do more than just run. Cross training can help to strengthen different groups of muscles, improve our coordination and build our aerobic capacity. It's not essential, but it's a great addition to a training plan. This is particularly the case if:

- You've been injured and need to return to running in a gradual way.
- You want or need to reduce the impact on your joints while still getting a good cardiovascular workout.
- Your menopausal barriers are making it hard to get out running whether that's breast pain, loss of running confidence or needing to be near a toilet.
- You feel stuck in a rut and want to mix things up.
- You've reached a running plateau or even lost your running mojo.
- It's not safe to run outside.

Find something that's convenient, a good workout and preferably fun. Cross training is a great way to maintain fitness if you can't run or don't want to run, for whatever reason.

GOOD TO KNOW

Treadmill running can be very helpful and I know people who have run successful marathons doing all their training on a treadmill. It's great if you want to run at a specific speed or set intervals or, of course, if the weather is bad or you don't want to head miles away from home. It's not quite the same as running outside, though, as the ground is pulled along underneath you and there is no air resistance, meaning you use less energy. To replicate outdoor running, set the gradient on the treadmill to 1 per cent for fast runs and 1 to 2 per cent for slower runs.

A SAMPLE WEEK

Let's look at a sample week of training. This is simply an idea for an average week when you aren't on any kind of training plan. Of course, everyone's week is different but here is a plan to fit in all the recommended activities when you want to do most of your running at the weekend. Warm up before each of these sessions and include a short cool-down too.

- Monday: Strength training and/or an easy run or cross training.
- Tuesday: Rest day and stretching.
- Wednesday: Sprint intervals.
- Thursday: Strength training with some plyometrics.
- Friday: Rest day.
- Saturday: Short run at whatever pace feels good on the day with some plyometrics.
- Sunday: Long, easy run.

The key is to be flexible and adjust your training to your schedule, but also to your energy levels on the day. You might be able to predict these according to what the week has in store for you, but they might be unpredictable thanks to hormone shifts. Stay open-minded, positive and self-aware. Never be afraid to take an extra rest day or do something completely different that just feels right for you. You know your running, your body and your menopause better than anyone, so be confident to make adaptations that suit you.

> 'My running is at a level I am happy with, and that my joints and energy levels can cope with. It's got a lot slower, but I find this is more enjoyable and kinder to my body.'
> **Sarah Jones,** Isle of Wight

CHAPTER 18

Training Plans

Some people think they aren't a real runner if they're not following a training plan and don't race, but running can be whatever you want it to be. Of course, you can just run intuitively whenever you like and if that's you – perhaps you're fairly new to running or you have no interest in entering events – just come back to this chapter if and when you're ready.

However, for women who do want to train for an event I've enlisted the help of Irene Clark, a running coach for peri- and post-menopausal women. She has created both half and full marathon plans for you, which take everything I've shared in this chapter into account. The plans are progressive and build slowly. They have rest days, step-back weeks, easy and interval runs, and strength work. These are tried and tested with groups of menopausal women, but they might look and feel different to training plans you're used to.

They're longer, and they ask for a good base of strength and aerobic capacity before you begin. Remember, you need to set yourself up to succeed and not to fail, and that looks different now you're in menopause. You're at more risk of injury and fatigue, and I want you to run healthily, so consider not signing up for that race right now and get the basics right first. When you're up to the level that Irene asks for, begin the plan, follow it as closely as you can and then go and run a really successful race. What many of us do is follow a plan we aren't ready for, push ourselves to perform on race day and then spend so long recovering from it that we lose the progress we've made. Clever, measured and flexible training is the key.

Meet the expert: Irene Clark

Irene has a background in sports science, and is a sports educator and coach specialising in menopause, endurance sports and participation sports. She works with active women of all levels, from recreational participants to competitive athletes, who share a common challenge: navigating the menopause years.

Her personal and professional experience led her to in-depth training and research on the science of midlife physiology, and how women can adapt to thrive, not just survive, during this stage of life.

In collaboration with Athletics Ireland, Irene developed and delivered the nationally recognised Mastering Midlife workshop for coaches and athletes, bridging the gap between hormonal health, training, nutrition and recovery. This was the first programme of its kind created for midlife women by any national governing body in Ireland. To date, over 5000 women have benefited from this initiative.

In addition, Irene leads the highly successful Reset Your Running programme and Mastering the Marathon in Midlife, Ireland's only menopause-specific marathon training programme.

Website: menopausecoach.ie, Instagram: menopause_coach_irene

WHICH PLAN SHOULD YOU CHOOSE?

Half marathon plans

- Level 1: Ideal if you're consistently running three times per week and have completed a 10km event.
- Level 2: Best if you're consistently running four times per week and have completed at least one half marathon.
- Level 3: Designed for runners logging 20 miles (32km) per week, running four times per week, who have completed multiple half marathons.

Marathon plans

- Level 1: Perfect if you're consistently running three times per week and have completed at least one half marathon.
- Level 2: Suitable for those running 25 miles (40km) per week, four times per week, who have completed at least one marathon.
- Level 3: Best for experienced marathoners running 30 miles (48km) per week, four times per week, who have completed multiple marathons.

HOW THE PLANS WORK

These training plans are designed to safely increase the distance you run while improving endurance and aerobic efficiency. Think of training plans like recipes – there are many ways to achieve great results using the same ingredients. With that in mind, and considering the unique challenges of training in midlife, these plans are designed as adaptable templates. While nothing can replace a personalised plan, the principles behind these templates will help guide you to both the start and finish line of your goal race.

The primary focus is aerobic training, which means a significant amount of easy running, which is one of the most valuable skills for long-term success. Many runners initially find themselves running at a slower pace than before. However, this doesn't mean you're losing speed, it means you're building a solid foundation for faster running in the future. Progress happens when your body adapts, not when you push beyond your limits. That's why every three weeks you'll have a step-back or recovery week, allowing your body to absorb the training and make real fitness gains.

A strong foundation determines your peak potential. Since a marathon is 99 per cent aerobic, maintaining a steady, low-intensity effort in zone 2 is crucial for long-term success. Even shorter races, like the 5km, are 84 per cent aerobic, emphasising the importance of a well-developed aerobic base.

Running faster than the prescribed effort shifts the workout's purpose, increases unnecessary stress on your body and raises the risk of injury. Discipline is key. Training at the right intensity is what drives real progress.

At a cellular level, meaningful adaptations take six to eight weeks, so trust the process. Your hard work will pay off and, when it does, you'll be ready to take your running to the next level.

GUIDELINES FOR ADAPTING YOUR PLAN

Stick to the plan: During the base training period, resist the urge to increase your distance. Your plan already includes plenty of volume and patience is key to long-term progress. The first few weeks will be conditioning weeks, prioritising low-intensity workouts to build a strong aerobic base. In your training plan, the session priority is listed with number 1 being the most important, 5 the least. If you need to drop a session, drop session 5.

Follow the hard/easy principle: Feel free to adjust sessions to fit your lifestyle, but never schedule two hard sessions back to back. Every intense workout should be followed by an easy day. The optimal training rhythm is three days of training, one rest day, two days of training, one rest day, ensuring recovery is spread throughout the week.

Take a step-back week every three weeks: As outlined in your plan, this week maintains workout intensity while reducing volume. Remember, all stress impacts your body, whether from training, work, family or menopause.

Pacing strategy: For easy runs, use heart rate as your guide. For faster sessions, focus on effort or pace.

Strength and conditioning: This is a crucial part of half and full marathon training. It's not optional, it's essential for keeping your body strong, resilient and injury free.

TYPES OF TRAINING RUNS

Long runs and easy runs

The main goal of long and easy runs is to build aerobic capacity and increase time on your feet. These runs should be kept at a maximum of zone 2 heart rate and if your heart rate stays below zone 2 that's perfectly fine. There's already plenty of training stimulus from your workouts throughout the week, so there's no need to push harder on these sessions.

Steady runs

Steady runs are slightly more challenging than easy runs and should be run at zone 3 heart rate. They provide a moderate intensity that bridges the gap between endurance-building and race-paced efforts.

Fartlek workout

After a warm-up and some strides, you'll run repetitions at a variety of different paces with jogging or walking to recover and allow your heart rate to lower.

Strides

Strides are fast but more controlled than an all-out sprint. After a warm-up, you'll do them over 60m with as much recovery as you need. They're included in some runs or as part of the warm-up for interval sessions.

Hill sprints

After a warm-up, you'll do some fast but relaxed strides to wake up your legs before the sprints. Then you'll head to a hill with a moderate incline (not too steep) and do fast sprints up the hill with a walk or slow jog down the hill to recover fully before the next sprint. Keep your eyes up towards the top of the hill to improve breathing and posture.

Hill repeats workout

Find a hill that is around 400m long with a moderate incline, steep enough to challenge you, but not so steep that it disrupts your form. After a warm-up and some strides, you'll be running with hard effort up and down the hill with an easy 400m recovery on the flat in between.

Interval runs

After at least a 10-minute warm-up of easy running, some strides will help transition to a faster pace. During the prescribed intervals, run at your current pace for the specified distance or time, rather than your goal pace for future races. There'll be jog recoveries between each interval. Treat the first interval as a warm-up and aim to finish feeling as though you could complete one or two more if needed.

Heart rate training zones

Training using heart rate zones is a more reliable and adaptable method than chasing specific paces. Heart rate training takes into account that many factors, such as fatigue, sleep, stress, menopause symptoms or even weather affect how fast you can run on any given day. By focusing on effort (via heart rate), you're ensuring consistency and reducing the risk of injury, since your body will be working at the right intensity, regardless of fluctuating pace.

Having a fitness tracker to measure heart rate makes this approach even more effective, as it helps you stay in the right zones. Your zones will be pre-set on your fitness tracker, so make sure you add your basic data, such as age and gender, to create appropriate zones for you.

Zone 1: 50–60% of max heart rate
This is a very light effort, mostly used for warm-ups, cool-downs or recovery runs. It's often called the 'active recovery' zone.

Zone 2: 60–70% of max heart rate
This is the key zone for building your aerobic base and endurance. You're running at a steady but sustainable pace. It's often called the 'aerobic zone', because it focuses on building cardiovascular efficiency and fat burning. Most of your training should occur here. Running too fast can quickly push you out of this zone and shift the focus from endurance to speed, which can hinder long-term progress.

Zone 3: 70–80% of max heart rate
This is a moderate effort, often referred to as the 'tempo' or 'threshold' zone. You can run here for extended periods, but it's more challenging than zone 2. It improves your ability to sustain faster efforts.

Zone 4: 80–90% of max heart rate
This is a hard effort, known as the 'lactate threshold' zone. Training in this zone boosts your speed and endurance at high intensities, but can only be maintained for shorter periods.

Zone 5: 90–100% of max heart rate
This is a maximal effort, used for short bursts (like sprints). It's focused on improving your power and speed.

Warm-ups and cool-downs

A warm-up has always been essential, but it becomes even more crucial as we age (see chapter 17). Cooling down is essential for initiating recovery, and since it can be more challenging for peri- and post-menopausal women to return to a resting state, an effective cool-down can assist with this process. The quicker we recover, the sooner we're ready for our next workout.

LEVEL 1 HALF MARATHON PLAN

Week	Focus	Day 1	Day 2	Day 3
1	Conditioning	Strength training • Priority 4 • 8/10 effort	Easy run with strides • Priority 3 • 3 miles (4.8km) • Warm up 15 mins, zone 2 • 4×60m strides with 60m jog recovery • Rest of run easy	Rest
2	Conditioning	Strength training • Priority 4 • 8/10 effort	Easy run with strides • Priority 3 • 3 miles (4.8km) • Warm up 15 mins, zone 2 • 4×60m strides with 60m jog recovery • Rest of run easy	Rest
3	Step back	Strength training • Priority 4 • 5/10 effort	Easy run with strides • Priority 3 • 3 miles (4.8km) • Warm up 15 mins, zone 2 • 4×60m strides with 60m jog recovery • Rest of run easy	Rest
4		Strength training • Priority 4 • 8/10 effort	Easy run with strides • Priority 3 • 3 miles (4.8km) • Warm up 15 mins, zone 2 • 4×60m strides with 60m jog recovery • Rest of run easy	Rest
5		Strength training • Priority 4 • 8/10 effort	Easy run with strides • Priority 3 • 3 miles (4.8km) • Warm up 15 mins, zone 2 • 4×60m strides with 60m jog recovery • Rest of run easy	Rest

Day 4	Day 5	Day 6	Day 7
Fartlek • Priority 2 • 3 miles (4.8km) • Warm up 15 mins, zone 2 • 4×60m strides with 60m jog recovery • 4–6×30 secs at mixed pace from 5km to marathon with 30 secs recovery • Rest of run easy	Strength training • Priority 5 • 8/10 effort	Long run • Priority 1 • 6 miles (9.6km) • Zone 2	Rest
Fartlek • Priority 2 • 4 miles (6.4km) • Warm up 15 mins, zone 2 • 4×60m strides with 60m jog recovery • 3–5×1 min at mixed pace from 5km to marathon with 1 min recovery • Rest of run easy	Strength training • Priority 5 • 8/10 effort	Long run • Priority 1 • 7 miles (11.2km) • Zone 2	Rest
Steady run • Priority 2 • 3 miles (4.8km) • Zone 3	Strength training • Priority 5 • 5/10 effort	Long run • Priority 1 • 5 miles (8km) • Zone 2	Rest
Fartlek • Priority 2 • 4 miles (6.4km) • Warm up 15 mins, zone 2 • 4×60m strides with 60m jog recovery • 2–4×1.5 min at mixed pace from 5km to marathon with 1.5 min recovery • Rest of run easy	Strength training • Priority 5 • 8/10 effort	Long run • Priority 1 • 8 miles (12.9km) • Zone 2	Rest
Fartlek • Priority 2 • 5 miles (8km) • Warm up 15 mins, zone 2 • 4×60m strides with 60m jog recovery • 2–3×2 mins at mixed pace from 5km to marathon with 2 min recovery • Rest of run easy	Strength training • Priority 5 • 8/10 effort	Long run • Priority 1 • 8 miles (12.9km) • Zone 2	Rest

Week	Focus	Day 1	Day 2	Day 3
6	Step back	Strength training • Priority 4 • 5/10 effort	Easy run with strides • Priority 3 • 3 miles (4.8km) • Warm up 15 mins, zone 2 • 4×60m strides with 60m jog recovery • Rest of run easy	Rest
7		Strength training • Priority 4 • 8/10 effort	Easy run with strides • Priority 3 • 3 miles (4.8km) • Warm up 15 mins, zone 2 • 6×60m strides with 60m jog recovery • Rest of run easy	Rest
8		Strength training • Priority 4 • 8/10 effort	Easy run with strides • Priority 3 • 3 miles (4.8km) • Warm up 15 mins, zone 2 • 6×60m strides with 60m jog recovery • Rest of run easy	Rest
9	Step back	Strength training • Priority 4 • 5/10 effort	Easy run with strides • Priority 3 • 3 miles (4.8km) • Warm up 15 mins, zone 2 • 6×60m strides with 60m jog recovery • Rest of run easy	Rest
10		Strength training • Priority 4 • 8/10 effort	Easy run with strides • Priority 3 • 4 miles (6.4km) • Warm up 15 mins, zone 2 • 6×60m strides with 60m jog recovery • Rest of run easy	Rest
11		Strength training • Priority 4 • 8/10 effort	Easy run with strides • Priority 3 • 4 miles (6.4km) • Warm up 15 mins, zone 2 • 6×60m strides with 60m jog recovery • Rest of run easy	Rest

Day 4	Day 5	Day 6	Day 7
Steady run • Priority 2 • 3 miles (4.8km) • Zone 3	Strength training • Priority 5 • 5/10 effort	Long run • Priority 1 • 6 miles (9.6km) • Zone 2	Rest
Hill sprints • Priority 2 • 5 miles (8km) • Warm up 15 mins, zone 2 • 4×60m strides with 60m jog recovery • 4×20 secs hard uphill, walk back down • Rest of run easy	Strength training • Priority 5 • 8/10 effort	Long run • Priority 1 • 9 miles (14.5km) • Zone 2	Rest
Hill sprints • Priority 2 • 5 miles (8km) • Warm up 15 mins, zone 2 • 4×60m strides with 60m jog recovery • 6×20 secs hard uphill, walk back down • Rest of run easy	Strength training • Priority 5 • 8/10 effort	Long run • Priority 1 • 10 miles (16km) • Zone 2	Rest
Steady run • Priority 2 • 4 miles (6.4km) • Zone 3	Strength training • Priority 5 • 5/10 effort	Long run • Priority 1 • 7 miles (11.2km) • Zone 2	Rest
Intervals • Priority 2 • 5 miles (8km) • Warm up 15 mins, zone 2 • 4×60m strides with 60m jog recovery • 2–3×3 mins at 5km effort with 3 min jog recovery • Rest of run easy	Strength training • Priority 5 • 8/10 effort	Long run • Priority 1 • 10 miles (16km) • Zone 2	Rest
Intervals • Priority 2 • 5 miles (8km) • Warm up 15 mins, zone 2 • 4×60m strides with 60m jog recovery • 2–3×4 mins at 5km effort with 4 min jog recovery • Rest of run easy	Strength training • Priority 5 • 8/10 effort	Long run • Priority 1 • 11 miles (17.7km) • Zone 2	Rest

Week	Focus	Day 1	Day 2	Day 3
12	Step back	Strength training • Priority 4 • 5/10 effort	Easy run with strides • Priority 3 • 4 miles (6.4km) • Warm up 15 mins, zone 2 • 6×60m strides with 60m jog recovery • Rest of run easy	Rest
13		Strength training • Priority 4 • 8/10 effort	Easy run with intervals • Priority 3 • 4 miles (6.4km) • Warm up 15 mins, zone 2 • 6×20 secs at 5km effort with 20 secs jog recovery • Rest of run easy	Rest
14		Strength training • Priority 4 • 8/10 effort	Easy run with intervals • Priority 3 • 3 miles (4.8km) • Warm up 15 mins, zone 2 • 4–5×30 secs at 5km effort with 30 secs jog recovery • Rest of run easy	Rest
15	Taper	Strength training • Priority 4 • 5/10 effort	Time trial • Priority 2 • 6 miles (9.6km) • Warm up 1 mile, zone 2 • 6×60m strides with 60m jog recovery • 5 miles at half marathon goal pace	Rest
16	Race week	Mobility training • Priority 4 • 3/10 effort	Easy run with strides and race pace • Priority 2 • 3 miles (4.8km) • Warm up 1 mile, zone 2 • 6×60m strides with 60m jog recovery • 2 miles at goal race pace	Rest

Day 4	Day 5	Day 6	Day 7
Steady run • Priority 2 • 4 miles (6.4km) • Zone 3	Strength training • Priority 5 • 5/10 effort	Long run • Priority 1 • 8 miles (12.9km) • Zone 2	Rest
Time trial • Priority 2 • 5 miles (8km) • Warm up 1 mile, zone 2 • 6×60m strides with 60m jog recovery • 5km at half marathon goal pace • 1 mile recovery	Strength training • Priority 5 • 8/10 effort	Long run • Priority 1 • 11 miles (17.7km) • Zone 2	Rest
Time trial • Priority 2 • 5 miles (8km) • Warm up 1 mile, zone 2 • 6×60m strides with 60m jog recovery • 4 miles at half marathon goal pace	Strength training • Priority 5 • 8/10 effort	Long run • Priority 1 • 12 miles (19.3km) • Zone 2	Rest
Easy run with strides • Priority 3 • 3 miles (4.8km) • Warm up 15 mins, zone 2 • 4×60m strides with 60m jog recovery • Rest of run easy	Strength training • Priority 5 • 5/10 effort	Long run • Priority 1 • 6 miles (9.6km) • Zone 2	Rest
Rest	Easy run with strides • Priority 3 • 2 miles (3.2km) • Warm up 15 mins, zone 2 • 6×60m strides with 60m jog recovery • Rest of run, zone 2	Half marathon • Priority 1 • 13.1 miles (21.1km) • Race pace	Rest

LEVEL 2 HALF MARATHON PLAN

Week	Focus	Day 1	Day 2	Day 3
1	Conditioning	Strength training • Priority 4 • 8/10 effort Easy run • Priority 4 • 3 miles (4.8km) • Zone 2	Easy run with strides • Priority 3 • 3 miles (4.8km) • Warm up 15 mins, zone 2 • 4×60m strides with 60m jog recovery • Rest of run easy	Rest
2	Conditioning	Strength training • Priority 4 • 8/10 effort Easy run • Priority 4 • 3 miles (4.8km) • Zone 2	Easy run with strides • Priority 3 • 3 miles (4.8km) • Warm up 15 mins, zone 2 • 4×60m strides with 60m jog recovery • Rest of run easy	Rest
3	Step back	Strength training • Priority 4 • 5/10 effort Easy run • Priority 4 • 3 miles (4.8km) • Zone 2	Easy run with strides • Priority 3 • 3 miles (4.8km) • Warm up 15 mins, zone 2 • 4×60m strides with 60m jog recovery • Rest of run easy	Rest
4		Strength training • Priority 4 • 8/10 effort Easy run • Priority 4 • 3 miles (4.8km) • Zone 2	Easy run with strides • Priority 3 • 4 miles (6.4km) • Warm up 15 mins, zone 2 • 4×60m strides with 60m jog recovery • Rest of run easy	Rest

Day 4	Day 5	Day 6	Day 7
Fartlek • Priority 2 • 4 miles (6.4km) • Warm up 15 mins, zone 2 • 4×60m strides with 60m jog recovery • 6–8×30 secs at mixed pace from 5km to marathon with 30 secs recovery • Rest of run easy	Strength training • Priority 5 • 8/10 effort	Long run • Priority 1 • 6 miles (9.6km) • Zone 2	Rest
Fartlek • Priority 2 • 5 miles (8km) • Warm up 15 mins, zone 2 • 4×60m strides with 60m jog recovery • 4–6×1 min at mixed pace from 5km to marathon with 1 min recovery • Rest of run easy	Strength training • Priority 5 • 8/10 effort	Long run • Priority 1 • 7 miles (11.2km) • Zone 2	Rest
Steady run • Priority 2 • 3 miles (4.8km) • Zone 3	Strength training • Priority 5 • 5/10 effort	Long run • Priority 1 • 5 miles (8km) • Zone 2	Rest
Fartlek • Priority 2 • 5 miles (8km) • Warm up 15 mins, zone 2 • 4×60m strides with 60m jog recovery • 3–5×1.5 min at mixed pace from 5km to marathon with 1.5 min recovery • Rest of run easy	Strength training • Priority 5 • 8/10 effort	Long run • Priority 1 • 8 miles (12.9km) • Zone 2	Rest

Week	Focus	Day 1	Day 2	Day 3
5		Strength training • Priority 4 • 8/10 effort Easy run • Priority 4 • 3 miles (4.8km) • Zone 2	Easy run with strides • Priority 3 • 4 miles (6.4km) • Warm up 15 mins, zone 2 • 4×60m strides with 60m jog recovery • Rest of run easy	Rest
6	Step back	Strength training • Priority 4 • 5/10 effort Easy run • Priority 4 • 3 miles (4.8km) • Zone 2	Easy run with strides • Priority 3 • 4 miles (6.4km) • Warm up 15 mins, zone 2 • 4×60m strides with 60m jog recovery • Rest of run easy	Rest
7		Strength training • Priority 4 • 8/10 effort Easy run • Priority 4 • 3 miles (4.8km) • Zone 2	Easy run with strides • Priority 3 • 4 miles (6.4km) • Warm up 15 mins, zone 2 • 6×60m strides with 60m jog recovery • Rest of run easy	Rest
8		Strength training • Priority 4 • 8/10 effort Easy run • Priority 4 • 3 miles (4.8km) • Zone 2	Easy run with strides • Priority 3 • 4 miles (6.4km) • Warm up 15 mins, zone 2 • 6×60m strides with 60m jog recovery • Rest of run easy	Rest
9	Step back	Strength training • Priority 4 • 5/10 effort Easy run • Priority 4 • 3 miles (4.8km) • Zone 2	Easy run with strides • Priority 3 • 4 miles (6.4km) • Warm up 15 mins, zone 2 • 6×60m strides with 60m jog recovery • Rest of run easy	Rest

Day 4	Day 5	Day 6	Day 7
Fartlek • Priority 2 • 5 miles (8km) • Warm up 15 mins, zone 2 • 4×60m strides with 60m jog recovery • 3–4×2 mins at mixed pace from 5km to marathon with 2 min recovery • Rest of run easy	Strength training • Priority 5 • 8/10 effort	Long run • Priority 1 • 9 miles (14.5km) • Zone 2	Rest
Steady run • Priority 2 • 3 miles (4.8km) • Zone 3	Strength training • Priority 5 • 5/10 effort	Long run • Priority 1 • 6 miles (9.6km) • Zone 2	Rest
Hill sprints • Priority 2 • 5 miles (8km) • Warm up 15 mins, zone 2 • 4×60m strides with 60m jog recovery • 4×30 secs hard uphill, walk back down • Rest of run easy	Strength training • Priority 5 • 8/10 effort	Long run • Priority 1 • 10 miles (16km) • Zone 2	Rest
Hill sprints • Priority 2 • 5 miles (8km) • Warm up 15 mins, zone 2 • 4×60m strides with 60m jog recovery • 4×30 secs hard uphill, walk back down • Rest of run easy	Strength training • Priority 5 • 8/10 effort	Long run • Priority 1 • 11 miles (17.7km) • Zone 2	Rest
Steady run • Priority 2 • 4 miles (6.4km) • Zone 3	Strength training • Priority 5 • 5/10 effort	Long run • Priority 1 • 7 miles (11.2km) • Zone 2	Rest

Week	Focus	Day 1	Day 2	Day 3
10		Strength training • Priority 4 • 8/10 effort Easy run • Priority 4 • 4 miles (6.4km) • Zone 2	Easy run with strides • Priority 3 • 4 miles (6.4km) • Warm up 15 mins, zone 2 • 6×60m strides with 60m jog recovery • Rest of run easy	Rest
11		Strength training • Priority 4 • 8/10 effort Easy run • Priority 4 • 3 miles (4.8km) • Zone 2	Easy run with strides • Priority 3 • 5 miles (8km) • Warm up 15 mins, zone 2 • 6×60m strides with 60m jog recovery • Rest of run easy	Rest
12	Step back	Strength training • Priority 4 • 5/10 effort Easy run • Priority 4 • 3 miles (4.8km) • Zone 2	Easy run with strides • Priority 3 • 4 miles (6.4km) • Warm up 15 mins, zone 2 • 6×60m strides with 60m jog recovery • Rest of run easy	Rest
13		Strength training • Priority 4 • 8/10 effort Easy run • Priority 4 • 4 miles (6.4km) • Zone 2	Easy run with intervals • Priority 3 • 4 miles (6.4km) • Warm up 15 mins, zone 2 • 6×30 secs at 5km effort with 30 secs jog recovery • Rest of run easy	Rest

Day 4	Day 5	Day 6	Day 7
Intervals • Priority 2 • 5 miles (8km) • Warm up 15 mins, zone 2 • 4×60m strides with 60m jog recovery • 3–4×3 mins at 5km effort with 3 min jog recovery • Rest of run easy	Strength training • Priority 5 • 8/10 effort	Long run • Priority 1 • 11 miles (17.7km) • Zone 2	Rest
Intervals • Priority 2 • 5 miles (8km) • Warm up 15 mins, zone 2 • 4×60m strides with 60m jog recovery • 3–4×4 mins at 5km effort with 4 min jog recovery • Rest of run easy	Strength training • Priority 5 • 8/10 effort	Long run • Priority 1 • 12 miles (19.3km) • Zone 2	Rest
Steady run • Priority 2 • 5 miles (8km) • Zone 3	Strength training • Priority 5 • 5/10 effort	Long run • Priority 1 • 7 miles (11.2km) • Zone 2	Rest
Time trial • Priority 2 • 5 miles (8km) • Warm up 1 mile, zone 2 • 6×60m strides with 60m jog recovery • 5km at half marathon goal pace • 1 mile recovery	Strength training • Priority 5 • 8/10 effort	Long run • Priority 1 • 12 miles (19.3km) • Zone 2	Rest

Week	Focus	Day 1	Day 2	Day 3
14		Strength training • Priority 4 • 8/10 effort Easy run • Priority 4 • 3 miles (4.8km) • Zone 2	Easy run with intervals • Priority 3 • 3 miles (4.8km) • Warm up 15 mins, zone 2 • 6×30 secs at 5km effort with 30 secs jog recovery • Rest of run easy	Rest
15	Taper	Strength training • Priority 4 • 5/10 effort	Time trial • Priority 2 • 7 miles (11.2km) • Warm up 1 mile, zone 2 • 6×60m strides with 60m jog recovery • 10K at half marathon goal pace	Rest
16	Race week	Mobility training • Priority 4 • 3/10 effort	Easy run with strides and race pace • Priority 2 • 4 miles (6.4km) • Warm up 1 mile, zone 2 • 6×60m strides with 60m jog recovery • 2 miles at goal race pace • Rest of run easy	Rest

LEVEL 3 HALF MARATHON PLAN

Week	Focus	Day 1	Day 2	Day 3
1	Conditioning	Strength training • Priority 4 • 8/10 effort Easy run • Priority 4 • 3 miles (4.8km) • Zone 2	Easy run with strides • Priority 3 • 4 miles (6.4km) • Warm up 15 mins, zone 2 • 4×60m strides with 60m jog recovery • Rest of run easy	Rest

Day 4	Day 5	Day 6	Day 7
Time trial • Priority 2 • 6 miles (9.6km) • Warm up 1 mile, zone 2 • 6×60m strides with 60m jog recovery • 5 miles at half marathon goal pace	Strength training • Priority 5 • 8/10 effort	Long run • Priority 1 • 13 miles (20.9km) • Zone 2	Rest
Easy run with strides • Priority 3 • 3 miles (4.8km) • Warm up 15 mins, zone 2 • 6×60m strides with 60m jog recovery • Rest of run easy	Strength training • Priority 5 • 5/10 effort	Long run • Priority 1 • 6 miles (9.6km) • Zone 2	Rest
Rest	Easy run with strides • Priority 3 • 2 miles (3.2km) • Warm up 15 mins, zone 2 • 6×60m strides with 60m jog recovery • Rest of run easy	Half marathon • Priority 1 • 13.1 miles (21.1km) • Race pace	Rest

Day 4	Day 5	Day 6	Day 7
Fartlek • Priority 2 • 5 miles (8km) • Warm up 15 mins, zone 2 • 4×60m strides with 60m jog recovery • 10×30 secs at mixed pace from 5km to marathon with 30 secs recovery • Rest of run easy	Strength training • Priority 5 • 8/10 effort	Long run • Priority 1 • 8 miles (12.9km) • Zone 2	Rest

Week	Focus	Day 1	Day 2	Day 3
2	Conditioning	Strength training • Priority 4 • 8/10 effort Easy run • Priority 4 • 3 miles (4.8km) • Zone 2	Easy run with strides • Priority 3 • 4 miles (6.4km) • Warm up 15 mins, zone 2 • 4×60m strides with 60m jog recovery • Rest of run easy	Rest
3	Step back	Strength training • Priority 4 • 5/10 effort Easy run • Priority 4 • 3 miles (4.8km) • Zone 2	Easy run with strides • Priority 3 • 3 miles (4.8km) • Warm up 15 mins, zone 2 • 4×60m strides with 60m jog recovery • Rest of run easy	Rest
4		Strength training • Priority 4 • 8/10 effort Easy run • Priority 4 • 3 miles (4.8km) • Zone 2	Easy run with strides • Priority 3 • 4 miles (6.4km) • Warm up 15 mins, zone 2 • 4×60m strides with 60m jog recovery • Rest of run easy	Rest
5		Strength training • Priority 4 • 8/10 effort Easy run • Priority 4 • 3 miles (4.8km) • Zone 2	Easy run with strides • Priority 3 • 5 miles (8km) • Warm up 15 mins, zone 2 • 4×60m strides with 60m jog recovery • Rest of run easy	Rest
6	Step back	Strength training • Priority 4 • 5/10 effort Easy run • Priority 4 • 3 miles (4.8km) • Zone 2	Easy run with strides • Priority 3 • 4 miles (6.4km) • Warm up 15 mins, zone 2 • 4×60m strides with 60m jog recovery • Rest of run easy	Rest

Day 4	Day 5	Day 6	Day 7
Fartlek • Priority 2 • 5 miles (8km) • Warm up 15 mins, zone 2 • 4×60m strides with 60m jog recovery • 7×1 min at mixed pace from 5km to marathon with 1 min recovery • Rest of run easy	Strength training • Priority 5 • 8/10 effort	Long run • Priority 1 • 9 miles (14.5km) • Zone 2	Rest
Steady run • Priority 2 • 4 miles (6.4km) • Zone 3	Strength training • Priority 5 • 5/10 effort	Long run • Priority 1 • 6 miles (9.6km) • Zone 2	Rest
Fartlek • Priority 2 • 6 miles (9.6km) • Warm up 15 mins, zone 2 • 4×60m strides with 60m jog recovery • 6×1.5 min at mixed pace from 5km to marathon with 1.5 min recovery • Rest of run easy	Strength training • Priority 5 • 8/10 effort	Long run • Priority 1 • 10 miles (16km) • Zone 2	Rest
Fartlek • Priority 2 • 6 miles (9.6km) • Warm up 15 mins, zone 2 • 4×60m strides with 60m jog recovery • 5×2 mins at mixed pace from 5km to marathon with 2 min recovery • Rest of run easy	Strength training • Priority 5 • 8/10 effort	Long run • Priority 1 • 11 miles (17.7km) • Zone 2	Rest
Steady run • Priority 2 • 5 miles (8km) • Zone 3	Strength training • Priority 5 • 5/10 effort	Long run • Priority 1 • 8 miles (12.9km) • Zone 2	Rest

Week	Focus	Day 1	Day 2	Day 3
7		Strength training • Priority 4 • 8/10 effort Easy run • Priority 4 • 3 miles (4.8km) • Zone 2	Easy run with strides • Priority 3 • 5 miles (8km) • Warm up 15 mins, zone 2 • 6×60m strides with 60m jog recovery • Rest of run easy	Rest
8		Strength training • Priority 4 • 8/10 effort Easy run • Priority 4 • 3 miles (4.8km) • Zone 2	Easy run with strides • Priority 3 • 6 miles (9.6km) • Warm up 15 mins, zone 2 • 6×60m strides with 60m jog recovery • Rest of run easy	Rest
9	Step back	Strength training • Priority 4 • 5/10 effort Easy run • Priority 4 • 3 miles (4.8km) • Zone 2	Easy run with strides • Priority 3 • 5 miles (8km) • Warm up 15 mins, zone 2 • 6×60m strides with 60m jog recovery • Rest of run easy	Rest
10		Strength training • Priority 4 • 8/10 effort Easy run • Priority 4 • 4 miles (6.4km) • Zone 2	Easy run with strides • Priority 3 • 6 miles (9.6km) • Warm up 15 mins, zone 2 • 6×60m strides with 60m jog recovery • Rest of run easy	Rest
11		Strength training • Priority 4 • 8/10 effort Easy run • Priority 4 • 4 miles (6.4km) • Zone 2	Easy run with strides • Priority 3 • 6 miles (9.6km) • Warm up 15 mins, zone 2 • 6×60m strides with 60m jog recovery • Rest of run easy	Rest

Day 4	Day 5	Day 6	Day 7
Hill sprints • Priority 2 • 6 miles (9.6km) • Warm up 15 mins, zone 2 • 4×60m strides with 60m jog recovery • 6×30 secs hard uphill, walk back down • Rest of run easy	Strength training • Priority 5 • 8/10 effort	Long run • Priority 1 • 12 miles (19.3km) • Zone 2	Rest
Hill sprints • Priority 2 • 6 miles (9.6km) • Warm up 15 mins, zone 2 • 4×60m strides with 60m jog recovery • 8×30 secs hard uphill, walk back down • Rest of run easy	Strength training • Priority 5 • 8/10 effort	Long run • Priority 1 • 12 miles (19.3km) • Zone 2	Rest
Steady run • Priority 2 • 5 miles (8km) • Zone 3	Strength training • Priority 5 • 5/10 effort	Long run • Priority 1 • 10 miles (16km) • Zone 2	Rest
Intervals • Priority 2 • 6 miles (9.6km) • Warm up 15 mins, zone 2 • 4×60m strides with 60m jog recovery • 6×3 mins at 5km effort with 3 min jog recovery • Rest of run easy	Strength training • Priority 5 • 8/10 effort	Long run • Priority 1 • 12 miles (19.3km) • Zone 2	Rest
Intervals • Priority 2 • 7 miles (11.2km) • Warm up 15 mins, zone 2 • 4×60m strides with 60m jog recovery • 5×4 mins at 5km effort with 4 min jog recovery • Rest of run easy	Strength training • Priority 5 • 8/10 effort	Long run • Priority 1 • 13 miles (20.9km) • Zone 2	Rest

Week	Focus	Day 1	Day 2	Day 3
12	Step back	Strength training • Priority 4 • 5/10 effort Easy run • Priority 4 • 3 miles (4.8km) • Zone 2	Easy run with strides • Priority 3 • 5 miles (8km) • Warm up 15 mins, zone 2 • 6×60m strides with 60m jog recovery • Rest of run easy	Rest
13		Strength training • Priority 4 • 8/10 effort Easy run • Priority 4 • 4 miles (6.4km) • Zone 2	Easy run with intervals • Priority 3 • 6 miles (9.6km) • Warm up 15 mins, zone 2 • 6×30 secs at 5km effort with 30 secs jog recovery • Rest of run easy	Rest
14		Strength training • Priority 4 • 8/10 effort Easy run • Priority 4 • 4 miles (6.4km) • Zone 2	Easy run with intervals • Priority 3 • 6 miles (9.6km) • Warm up 15 mins, zone 2 • 6×30 secs at 5km effort with 30 secs jog recovery • Rest of run easy	Rest
15	Taper	Strength training • Priority 4 • 5/10 effort Easy run • Priority 4 • 3 miles (4.8km) • Zone 2	Time trial • Priority 2 • 7 miles (11.2km) • Warm up 1 mile, zone 2 • 6×60m strides with 60m jog recovery • 10km at half marathon goal pace	Rest
16	Race week	Mobility training • Priority 4 • 3/10 effort	Easy run with strides and race pace • Priority 2 • 5 miles (8km) • Warm up 2 miles, zone 2 • 6×60m strides with 60m jog recovery • 2 miles at goal race pace • Rest of run easy	Rest

Day 4	Day 5	Day 6	Day 7
Steady run • Priority 2 • 6 miles (9.6km) • Zone 3	Strength training • Priority 5 • 5/10 effort	Long run • Priority 1 • 10 miles (16km) • Zone 2	Rest
Time trial • Priority 2 • 7 miles (11.2km) • Warm up 2 miles, zone 2 • 6×60m strides with 60m jog recovery • 5km at half marathon goal pace • 2 miles recovery	Strength training • Priority 5 • 8/10 effort	Long run • Priority 1 • 13 miles (20.9km) • Zone 2	Rest
Time trial • Priority 2 • 7 miles (11.2km) • Warm up 2 miles, zone 2 • 6×60m strides with 60m jog recovery • 5 miles at half marathon goal pace	Strength training • Priority 5 • 8/10 effort	Long run • Priority 1 • 12 miles (19.3km) • Zone 2	Rest
Easy run with strides • Priority 3 • 4 miles (6.4km) • Warm up 15 mins, zone 2 • 6×60m strides with 60m jog recovery • Rest of run easy	Strength training • Priority 5 • 5/10 effort	Long run • Priority 1 • 6 miles (9.6km) • Zone 2	Rest
Rest	Easy run with strides • Priority 3 • 2 miles (3.2km) • Warm up 15 mins, zone 2 • 6×60m strides with 60m jog recovery • Rest of run easy	Half marathon • Priority 1 • 13.1 miles (21.1km) • Race pace	Rest

LEVEL 1 MARATHON PLAN

Week	Focus	Day 1	Day 2	Day 3
1	Conditioning	Strength training • Priority 4 • 8/10 effort	Easy run with strides • Priority 3 • 6 miles (9.6km) • Warm up 15 mins, zone 2 • 4×60m strides with 60m jog recovery • Rest of run easy	Rest
2	Conditioning	Strength training • Priority 4 • 8/10 effort	Easy run with strides • Priority 3 • 6 miles (9.6km) • Warm up 15 mins, zone 2 • 6×60m strides with 60m jog recovery • Rest of run easy	Rest
3	Step back	Strength training • Priority 4 • 5/10 effort	Easy run with strides • Priority 3 • 4 miles (6.4km) • Warm up 15 mins, zone 2 • 4×60m strides with 60m jog recovery • Rest of run easy	Rest
4		Strength training • Priority 4 • 8/10 effort	Easy run with strides • Priority 3 • 6 miles (9.6km) • Warm up 15 mins, zone 2 • 6×60m strides with 60m jog recovery • Rest of run easy	Rest

Day 4	Day 5	Day 6	Day 7
Fartlek • Priority 2 • 6 miles (9.6km) • Warm up 15 mins, zone 2 • 4×60m strides with 60m jog recovery • 4–6×30 secs at mixed pace from 5km to marathon with 30 secs recovery • Rest of run easy	Strength training/cross train • Priority 5 • 8/10 effort • Zone 1–2 for 30 mins	Long run • Priority 1 • 8 miles (12.9km) • Zone 2	Rest
Fartlek • Priority 2 • 6 miles (9.6km) • Warm up 15 mins, zone 2 • 4×60m strides with 60m jog recovery • 3–4×1 min at mixed pace from 5km to marathon with 1 min recovery • Rest of run easy	Strength training/cross train • Priority 5 • 8/10 effort • Zone 1–2 for 30 mins	Long run • Priority 1 • 9 miles (14.5km) • Zone 2	Rest
Steady run • Priority 2 • 5 miles (8km) • 5/10 effort	Strength training/cross train • Priority 5 • 5/10 effort • Zone 1–2 for 30 mins	Long run • Priority 1 • 8 miles (12.9km) • Zone 2	Rest
Fartlek • Priority 2 • 6 miles (9.6km) • Warm up 15 mins, zone 2 • 4×60m strides with 60m jog recovery • 2–4×1.5 min at mixed pace from 5km to marathon with 1.5 min recovery • Rest of run easy	Strength training/cross train • Priority 5 • 8/10 effort • Zone 1–2 for 30 mins	Long run • Priority 1 • 11 miles (17.7km) • Zone 2	Rest

Week	Focus	Day 1	Day 2	Day 3
5		Strength training • Priority 4 • 8/10 effort	Easy run with strides • Priority 3 • 6 miles (9.6km) • Warm up 15 mins, zone 2 • 8×60m strides with 60m jog recovery • Rest of run easy	Rest
6	Step back	Strength training • Priority 4 • 5/10 effort	Easy run with strides • Priority 3 • 4 miles (6.4km) • Warm up 15 mins, zone 2 • 4×60m strides with 60m jog recovery • Rest of run easy	Rest
7		Strength training • Priority 4 • 8/10 effort	Easy run with strides • Priority 3 • 6 miles (9.6km) • Warm up 15 mins, zone 2 • 6×60m strides with 60m jog recovery • Rest of run easy	Rest
8		Strength training • Priority 4 • 8/10 effort	Easy run with strides • Priority 3 • 6 miles (9.6km) • Warm up 15 mins, zone 2 • 8×60m strides with 60m jog recovery • Rest of run easy	Rest

Day 4	Day 5	Day 6	Day 7
Fartlek - Priority 2 - 6 miles (9.6km) - Warm up 15 mins, zone 2 - 4×60m strides with 60m jog recovery - 2–3×2 mins at mixed pace from 5km to marathon with 2 min recovery - Rest of run easy	Strength training/cross train - Priority 5 - 8/10 effort - Zone 1–2 for 30 mins	Long run - Priority 1 - 12 miles (19.3km) - Zone 2	Rest
Steady run - Priority 2 - 5 miles (8km) - Zone 3	Strength training/cross train - Priority 5 - 5/10 effort - Zone 1–2 for 30 mins	Long run - Priority 1 - 9 miles (14.5km) - Zone 2	Rest
Fartlek - Priority 2 - 6 miles (9.6km) - Warm up 15 mins, zone 2 - 4×60m strides with 60m jog recovery - 1–2×4 mins at mixed pace from 10-mile to half marathon pace with 2 min recovery - Rest of run easy	Strength training/cross train - Priority 5 - 8/10 effort - Zone 1–2 for 30 mins	Long run - Priority 1 - 13 miles (20.9km) - Zone 2	Rest
Fartlek - Priority 2 - 6 miles (9.6km) - Warm up 15 mins, zone 2 - 4×60m strides with 60m jog recovery - 1–2×6 mins at mixed pace from 10-mile to half marathon pace with 3 min recovery - Rest of run easy	Strength training/cross train - Priority 5 - 8/10 effort - Zone 1–2 for 30 mins	Long run - Priority 1 - 14 miles (22.5km) - Zone 2	Rest

Week	Focus	Day 1	Day 2	Day 3
9	Step back	Strength training • Priority 4 • 5/10 effort	Hill sprints • Priority 3 • 4 miles (6.4km) • Warm up 15 mins, zone 2 • 4×60m strides with 60m jog recovery • 4–6×15 secs hard uphill and walk back down • Rest of run easy	Rest
10		Strength training • Priority 4 • 8/10 effort	Hill sprints • Priority 3 • 7 miles (11.2km) • Warm up 15 mins, zone 2 • 4×60m strides with 60m jog recovery • 3–4×20 secs hard uphill and walk back down • Rest of run easy	Rest
11		Strength training • Priority 4 • 8/10 effort	Hill sprints • Priority 3 • 6 miles (9.6km) • Warm up 15 mins, zone 2 • 4×60m strides with 60m jog recovery • 4×30 secs hard uphill and walk back down • Rest of run easy	Rest
12	Step back	Strength training • Priority 4 • 5/10 effort	Hill repeats • Priority 2 • 6 miles (9.6km) • Warm up 15 mins, zone 2 • 4×60m strides with 60m jog recovery • 400m easy, 400m hard uphill, 400m easy, 400m hard downhill (two sets) • Rest of run easy	Rest

Day 4	Day 5	Day 6	Day 7
Steady run • Priority 2 • 6 miles (9.6km) • Zone 3	Strength training/cross train • Priority 5 • 5/10 effort • Zone 1–2 for 30 mins	Long run • Priority 1 • 10 miles (16km) • Zone 2	Rest
Hill repeats • Priority 2 • 6 miles (9.6km) • Warm up 15 mins, zone 2 • 4×60m strides with 60m jog recovery • 400m easy, 400m hard uphill, 400m easy, 400m hard downhill (1 set) • Rest of run easy	Strength training/cross train • Priority 5 • 8/10 effort • Zone 1–2 for 30 mins	Long run • Priority 1 • 14 miles (22.5km) • Zone 2	Rest
Hill repeats • Priority 2 • 7 miles (11.2km) • Warm up 15 mins, zone 2 • 4×60m strides with 60m jog recovery • 400m easy, 400m hard uphill, 400m easy, 400m hard downhill (two sets) • Rest of run easy	Strength training/cross train • Priority 5 • 8/10 effort • Zone 1–2 for 30 mins	Long run • Priority 1 • 15 miles (24.1km) • Zone 2	Rest
Easy run with strides • Priority 3 • 4 miles (6.4km) • Warm up 15 mins, zone 2 • 6×60m strides with 60m jog recovery • Rest of run easy	Strength training/cross train • Priority 5 • 5/10 effort • Zone 1–2 for 30 mins	Long run • Priority 1 • 13 miles (20.9km) • Zone 2	Rest

Week	Focus	Day 1	Day 2	Day 3
13		Strength training • Priority 4 • 8/10 effort	Easy run with intervals • Priority 3 • 6 miles (9.6km) • Warm up 15 mins, zone 2 • 4–5×30 secs at 5km effort with 30 secs jog recovery • Rest of run easy	Rest
14		Strength training • Priority 4 • 8/10 effort	Easy run with intervals • Priority 3 • 6 miles (9.6km) • Warm up 15 mins, zone 2 • 2–3×30 secs at 5km effort with 30 secs jog recovery • Rest of run easy	Rest
15	Step back	Strength training • Priority 4 • 5/10 effort	Easy run with strides and race pace • Priority 2 • 4 miles (6.4km) • Warm up 15 mins, zone 2 • 4×60m strides with 60m jog recovery • 2 miles at half marathon pace • Rest of run easy	Rest
16		Strength training • Priority 4 • 8/10 effort	Easy run with intervals • Priority 3 • 7 miles (11.2km) • Warm up 15 mins, zone 2 • 2–3×30 secs at 5km effort with 30 secs jog recovery • Rest of run easy	Rest

Day 4	Day 5	Day 6	Day 7
Intervals • Priority 2 • 7 miles (11.2km) • Warm up 2 miles, zone 2 • 6×60m strides with 60m jog recovery • 3–4×2 mins at 5km effort with 2 min jog recovery • Rest of run easy	Strength training/cross train • Priority 5 • 8/10 effort • Zone 1–2 for 30 mins	Long run • Priority 1 • 16 miles (25.7km) • Zone 2 with last 6 miles at marathon pace	Rest
Intervals • Priority 2 • 7 miles (11.2km) • Warm up 2 miles, zone 2 • 6×60m strides with 60m jog recovery • 3–4×3 mins at 5km effort with 4 min jog recovery • Rest of run easy	Strength training/cross train • Priority 5 • 8/10 effort • Zone 1–2 for 30 mins	Long run • Priority 1 • 17 miles (27.3km) • Zone 2	Rest
Mobility training • Priority 5 • 3/10 effort	Easy run with strides • Priority 3 • 2 miles (3.2km) • Warm up 15 mins, zone 2 • 4×60m strides with 60m jog recovery • Rest of run easy	Half marathon race • Priority 1 • 13.1 miles (21.1km)	Rest
Intervals • Priority 2 • 7 miles (11.2km) • Warm up 2 miles, zone 2 • 6×60m strides with 60m jog recovery • 2–3×4 mins at 5km effort with 6 min jog recovery • Rest of run easy	Strength training/cross train • Priority 5 • 8/10 effort • Zone 1–2 for 30 mins	Long run • Priority 1 • 18 miles (29km) • Zone 2	Rest

Week	Focus	Day 1	Day 2	Day 3
17		Strength training • Priority 4 • 8/10 effort	Easy run with intervals • Priority 3 • 8 miles (12.9km) • Warm up 15 mins, zone 2 • 2–3×30 secs at 5km effort with 30 secs jog recovery • Rest of run easy	Rest
18	Taper	Strength training • Priority 4 • 5/10 effort	Intervals • Priority 2 • 6 miles (9.6km) • Warm up 2 miles, zone 2 • 6×60m strides with 60m jog recovery • 3–4mins at 5km effort with 4 min jog recovery • Rest of run easy	Rest
19	Taper	Strength training • Priority 4 • 5/10 effort	Time trial • Priority 2 • 6 miles (9.6km) at marathon pace	Rest
20	Race week	Mobility training • Priority 4 • 3/10 effort	Easy run with strides and race pace • Priority 2 • 4 miles (6.4km) • Warm up 1 mile, zone 2 • 6×60m strides with 60m jog recovery • 2 miles at goal race pace • Rest of run easy	Rest

Day 4	Day 5	Day 6	Day 7
Intervals • Priority 2 • 7 miles (11.2km) • Warm up 2 miles, zone 2 • 6×60m strides with 60m jog recovery • 2×800m at 5km effort with 5 min jog recovery • Rest of run easy	Strength training/cross train • Priority 5 • 8/10 effort • Zone 1–2 for 30 mins	Long run • Priority 1 • 18 miles (29km) • Zone 2 with last 8 miles at marathon pace	Rest
Easy run with strides • Priority 3 • 6 miles (9.6km) • Warm up 15 mins, zone 2 • 4×60m strides with 60m jog recovery • Rest of run easy	Strength training/cross train • Priority 5 • 5/10 effort • Zone 1–2 for 30 mins	Long run • Priority 1 • 13 miles (20.9km) • Zone 2	Rest
Easy run with strides • Priority 3 • 4 miles (6.4km) • Warm up 15 mins, zone 2 • 4×60m strides with 60m jog recovery • Rest of run easy	Strength training • Priority 5 • 5/10 effort	Long run • Priority 1 • 10 miles (16km) • Zone 2	Rest
Rest	Easy run with strides • Priority 3 • 2 miles (3.2km) • Warm up 15 mins, zone 2 • 6×60m strides with 60m jog recovery • Rest of run easy	Marathon race • Priority 1 • 26.2 miles (42.2km) • Race pace	Rest

LEVEL 2 MARATHON PLAN

Week	Focus	Day 1	Day 2	Day 3
1	Conditioning	Strength training • Priority 4 • 8/10 effort Easy run • Priority 4 • 4 miles (6.4km) • Zone 2	Easy run with strides • Priority 3 • 6 miles (9.6km) • Warm up 15 mins, zone 2 • 4×60m strides with 60m jog recovery • Rest of run easy	Rest
2	Conditioning	Strength training • Priority 4 • 8/10 effort Easy run • Priority 4 • 3 miles (4.8km) • Zone 2	Easy run with strides • Priority 3 • 7 miles (11.2km) • Warm up 15 mins, zone 2 • 6×60m strides with 60m jog recovery • Rest of run easy	Rest
3	Step back	Strength training • Priority 4 • 5/10 effort Easy run • Priority 4 • 3 miles (4.8km) • Zone 2	Easy run with strides • Priority 3 • 4 miles (6.4km) • Warm up 15 mins, zone 2 • 4×60m strides with 60m jog recovery • Rest of run easy	Rest
4		Strength training • Priority 4 • 8/10 effort Easy run • Priority 4 • 3 miles (4.8km) • Zone 2	Easy run with strides • Priority 3 • 7 miles (11.2km) • Warm up 15 mins, zone 2 • 6×60m strides with 60m jog recovery • Rest of run easy	Rest

Day 4	Day 5	Day 6	Day 7
Fartlek • Priority 2 • 5 miles (8km) • Warm up 15 mins, zone 2 • 4×60m strides with 60m jog recovery • 6–8×30 secs at mixed pace from 5km to marathon with 30 secs recovery • Rest of run easy	Strength training/ cross train • Priority 5 • 8/10 effort • Zone 1–2 for 30 mins	Long run • Priority 1 • 10 miles (16km) • Zone 2	Rest
Fartlek • Priority 2 • 5 miles (8km) • Warm up 15 mins, zone 2 • 4×60m strides with 60m jog recovery • 4–6×1 min at mixed pace from 5km to marathon with 1 min recovery • Rest of run easy	Strength training/ cross train • Priority 5 • 8/10 effort • Zone 1–2 for 30 mins	Long run • Priority 1 • 12 miles (19.3km) • Zone 2	Rest
Steady run • Priority 2 • 5 miles (8km) • Zone 3	Strength training/ cross train • Priority 5 • 5/10 effort • Zone 1–2 for 30 mins	Long run • Priority 1 • 8 miles (12.9km) • Zone 2	Rest
Fartlek • Priority 2 • 6 miles (9.6km) • Warm up 15 mins, zone 2 • 4×60m strides with 60m jog recovery • 3–5×1.5 min at mixed pace from 5km to marathon with 1.5 min recovery • Rest of run easy	Strength training/ cross train • Priority 5 • 8/10 effort • Zone 1–2 for 30 mins	Long run • Priority 1 • 12 miles (19.3km) • Zone 2	Rest

Week	Focus	Day 1	Day 2	Day 3
5		Strength training • Priority 4 • 8/10 effort Easy run • Priority 4 • 3 miles (4.8km) • Zone 2	Easy run with strides • Priority 3 • 8 miles (12.9km) • Warm up 15 mins, zone 2 • 8×60m strides with 60m jog recovery • Rest of run easy	Rest
6	Step back	Strength training • Priority 4 • 5/10 effort Easy run • Priority 4 • 3 miles (4.8km) • Zone 2	Easy run with strides • Priority 3 • 4 miles (6.4km) • Warm up 15 mins, zone 2 • 4×60m strides with 60m jog recovery • Rest of run easy	Rest
7		Strength training • Priority 4 • 8/10 effort Easy run • Priority 4 • 3 miles (4.8km) • Zone 2	Easy run with strides • Priority 3 • 9 miles (14.5km) • Warm up 15 mins, zone 2 • 8×60m strides with 60m jog recovery • Rest of run easy	Rest
8		Strength training • Priority 4 • 8/10 effort Easy run • Priority 4 • 3 miles (4.8km) • Zone 2	Easy run with strides • Priority 3 • 10 miles (16km) • Warm up 15 mins, zone 2 • 8×60m strides with 60m jog recovery • Rest of run easy	Rest

Day 4	Day 5	Day 6	Day 7
Fartlek • Priority 2 • 6 miles (9.6km) • Warm up 15 mins, zone 2 • 4×60m strides with 60m jog recovery • 2-4×2 mins at mixed pace from 5km to marathon with 2 min recovery • Rest of run easy	Strength training/cross train • Priority 5 • 8/10 effort • Zone 1-2 for 30 mins	Long run • Priority 1 • 13 miles (20.9km) • Zone 2	Rest
Steady run • Priority 2 • 5 miles (8km) • Zone 3	Strength training/cross train • Priority 5 • 5/10 effort • Zone 1-2 for 30 mins	Long run • Priority 1 • 9 miles (14.5km) • Zone 2	Rest
Fartlek • Priority 2 • 6 miles (9.6km) • Warm up 15 mins, zone 2 • 4×60m strides with 60m jog recovery • 2-3×4 mins at mixed pace from 10-mile to half marathon pace with 2 min recovery • Rest of run easy	Strength training/cross train • Priority 5 • 8/10 effort • Zone 1-2 for 30 mins	Long run • Priority 1 • 13 miles (20.9km) • Zone 2	Rest
Fartlek • Priority 2 • 6 miles (9.6km) • Warm up 15 mins, zone 2 • 4×60m strides with 60m jog recovery • 1-2×8 mins at mixed pace from 10-mile to half marathon pace with 3 min recovery • Rest of run easy	Strength training/cross train • Priority 5 • 8/10 effort • Zone 1-2 for 30 mins	Long run • Priority 1 • 14 miles (22.5km) • Zone 2	Rest

Week	Focus	Day 1	Day 2	Day 3
9	Step back	Strength training • Priority 4 • 5/10 effort Easy run • Priority 4 • 3 miles (4.8km) • Zone 2	Hill sprints • Priority 3 • 4 miles (6.4km) • Warm up 15 mins, zone 2 • 4×60m strides with 60m jog recovery • 4–6×15 secs hard uphill and walk back down • Rest of run easy	Rest
10		Strength training • Priority 4 • 8/10 effort Easy run • Priority 4 • 4 miles (6.4km) • Zone 2	Hill sprints • Priority 3 • 10 miles (16km) • Warm up 15 mins, zone 2 • 4×60m strides with 60m jog recovery • 4–6×20 secs hard uphill and walk back down • Rest of run easy	Rest
11		Strength training • Priority 4 • 8/10 effort Easy run • Priority 4 • 4 miles (6.4km) • Zone 2	Hill sprints • Priority 3 • 10 miles (16km) • Warm up 15 mins, zone 2 • 4×60m strides with 60m jog recovery • 6×30 secs hard uphill and walk back down • Rest of run easy	Rest
12	Step back	Strength training • Priority 4 • 5/10 effort Easy run • Priority 4 • 3 miles (4.8km) • Zone 2	Hill repeats • Priority 2 • 6 miles (9.6km) • Warm up 15 mins, zone 2 • 4×60m strides with 60m jog recovery • 400m easy, 400m hard uphill, 400m easy, 400m hard downhill (three sets) • Rest of run easy	Rest

Day 4	Day 5	Day 6	Day 7
Steady run • Priority 2 • 6 miles (9.6km) • Zone 3	Strength training/ cross train • Priority 5 • 5/10 effort • Zone 1–2 for 30 mins	Long run • Priority 1 • 10 miles (16km) • Zone 2	Rest
Hill repeats • Priority 2 • 6 miles (9.6km) • Warm up 15 mins, zone 2 • 4×60m strides with 60m jog recovery • 400m easy, 400m hard uphill, 400m easy, 400m hard downhill (1 set) • Rest of run easy	Strength training/ cross train • Priority 5 • 8/10 effort • Zone 1–2 for 30 mins	Long run • Priority 1 • 14 miles (22.5km) • Zone 2	Rest
Hill repeats • Priority 2 • 7 miles (11.2km) • Warm up 15 mins, zone 2 • 4×60m strides with 60m jog recovery • 400m easy, 400m hard uphill, 400m easy, 400m hard downhill (two sets) • Rest of run easy	Strength training/ cross train • Priority 5 • 8/10 effort • Zone 1–2 for 30 mins	Long run • Priority 1 • 15 miles (24.1km) • Zone 2	Rest
Easy run with strides • Priority 3 • 4 miles (6.4km) • Warm up 15 mins, zone 2 • 8×60m strides with 60m jog recovery • Rest of run easy	Strength training/ cross train • Priority 5 • 5/10 effort • Zone 1–2 for 30 mins	Long run • Priority 1 • 13 miles (20.9km) • Zone 2	Rest

Week	Focus	Day 1	Day 2	Day 3
13		Strength training • Priority 4 • 8/10 effort Easy run • Priority 4 • 4 miles (6.4km) • Zone 2	Easy run with intervals • Priority 3 • 10 miles (16km) • Warm up 15 mins, zone 2 • 4–5×30 secs at 5km effort with 30 secs jog recovery • Rest of run easy	Rest
14		Strength training • Priority 4 • 8/10 effort Easy run • Priority 4 • 4 miles (6.4km) • Zone 2	Easy run with intervals • Priority 3 • 10 miles (16km) • Warm up 15 mins, zone 2 • 4–5×30 secs at 5km effort with 30 secs jog recovery • Rest of run easy	Rest
15	Step back	Strength training • Priority 4 • 5/10 effort Easy run • Priority 4 • 3 miles (4.8km) • Zone 2	Easy run with strides and race pace • Priority 2 • 4 miles (6.4km) • Warm up 15 mins, zone 2 • 6×60m strides with 60m jog recovery • 2 miles at half marathon pace • Rest of run easy	Rest
16		Strength training • Priority 4 • 3/10 effort Easy run • Priority 4 • 4 miles (6.4km) • Zone 2	Easy run with intervals • Priority 3 • 7 miles (11.2km) • Warm up 15 mins, zone 2 • 4–5×30 secs at 5km effort with 30 secs jog recovery • Rest of run easy	Rest
17		Strength training • Priority 4 • 8/10 effort Easy run • Priority 4 • 4 miles (6.4km) • Zone 2	Easy run with intervals • Priority 3 • 10 miles (16km) • Warm up 15 mins, zone 2 • 4–5×30 secs at 5km effort with 30 secs jog recovery • Rest of run easy	Rest

Day 4	Day 5	Day 6	Day 7
Intervals • Priority 2 • 7 miles (11.2km) • Warm up 2 miles, zone 2 • 6×60m strides with 60m jog recovery • 4–6×2 mins at 5km effort with 2 min jog recovery • Rest of run easy	Strength training/cross train • Priority 5 • 8/10 effort • Zone 1–2 for 30 mins	Long run • Priority 1 • 16 miles (25.7km) • Zone 2 with last 6 miles at marathon pace	Rest
Intervals • Priority 2 • 7 miles (11.2km) • Warm up 2 miles, zone 2 • 6×60m strides with 60m jog recovery • 4–5×3 mins at 5km effort with 4 min jog recovery • Rest of run easy	Strength training/cross train • Priority 5 • 8/10 effort • Zone 1–2 for 30 mins	Long run • Priority 1 • 17 miles (27.3km) • Zone 2	Rest
Mobility training • Priority 5 • 3/10 effort	Easy run with strides • Priority 3 • 2 miles (3.2km) • Warm up 15 mins, zone 2 • 4×60m strides with 60m jog recovery • Rest of run easy	Half marathon race • Priority 1 • 13.1 miles (21.1km)	Rest
Intervals • Priority 2 • 10 miles (16km) • Warm up 2 miles, zone 2 • 6×60m strides with 60m jog recovery • 2–3×6 mins at 5km effort with 6 min jog recovery • Rest of run easy	Strength training/cross train • Priority 5 • 8/10 effort • Zone 1–2 for 30 mins	Long run • Priority 1 • 18 miles (29km) • Zone 2	Rest
Intervals • Priority 2 • 7 miles (11.2km) • Warm up 2 miles, zone 2 • 6×60m strides with 60m jog recovery • 2–3×800m at 5km effort with 5 min jog recovery • Rest of run easy	Strength training/cross train • Priority 5 • 8/10 effort • Zone 1–2 for 30 mins	Long run • Priority 1 • 19 miles (30.5km) • Zone 2 with last 8 miles at marathon pace	Rest

Week	Focus	Day 1	Day 2	Day 3
18	Taper	Strength training • Priority 4 • 5/10 effort Easy run • Priority 4 • 3 miles (4.8km) • Zone 2	Intervals • Priority 2 • 7 miles (11.2km) • Warm up 2 miles, zone 2 • 6×60m strides with 60m jog recovery • 4–6×4mins at 5km effort with 4 min jog recovery • Rest of run easy	Rest
19	Taper	Strength training • Priority 4 • 5/10 effort Easy run • Priority 4 • 3 miles (4.8km) • Zone 2	Time trial • Priority 2 • 6 miles (9.6km) at marathon pace	Rest
20	Race week	Mobility training • Priority 4 • 3/10 effort	Easy run with strides and race pace • Priority 2 • 5 miles (8km) • Warm up 2 miles zone 2 • 6×60m strides with 60m jog recovery • 2 miles at goal race pace • Rest of run easy	Rest

LEVEL 3 MARATHON PLAN

Week	Focus	Day 1	Day 2	Day 3
1	Conditioning	Strength training • Priority 4 • 8/10 effort Easy run • Priority 4 • 6 miles (9.6km) • Zone 2	Easy run with strides • Priority 3 • 6 miles (9.6km) • Warm up 15 mins, zone 2 • 4×60m strides with 60m jog recovery • Rest of run easy	Rest

Day 4	Day 5	Day 6	Day 7
Easy run with strides • Priority 3 • 5 miles (8km) • Warm up 15 mins, zone 2 • 6×60m strides with 60m jog recovery • Rest of run easy	Strength training/cross train • Priority 5 • 5/10 effort • Zone 1–2 for 30 mins	Long run • Priority 1 • 14 miles (22.5km) • Zone 2	Rest
Easy run with strides • Priority 3 • 4 miles (6.4km) • Warm up 15 mins, zone 2 • 6×60m strides with 60m jog recovery • Rest of run easy	Strength training • Priority 5 • 5/10 effort	Long run • Priority 1 • 10 miles (16km) • Zone 2	Rest
Rest	Easy run with strides • Priority 3 • 2 miles (3.2km) • Warm up 15 mins, zone 2 • 6×60m strides with 60m jog recovery • Rest of run easy	Marathon race • Priority 1 • 26.2 miles (42.2km) • Race pace	Rest

Day 4	Day 5	Day 6	Day 7
Fartlek • Priority 2 • 6 miles (9.6km) • Warm up 15 mins, zone 2 • 4×60m strides with 60m jog recovery • 10×30 secs at mixed pace from 5km to marathon with 30 secs recovery • Rest of run easy	Strength training/cross train • Priority 5 • 8/10 effort • Zone 1–2 for 30 mins	Long run • Priority 1 • 12 miles (19.3km) • Zone 2	Rest

Week	Focus	Day 1	Day 2	Day 3
2	Conditioning	Strength training • Priority 4 • 8/10 effort Easy run • Priority 4 • 6 miles (9.6km) • Zone 2	Easy run with strides • Priority 3 • 7 miles (11.2km) • Warm up 15 mins, zone 2 • 6×60m strides with 60m jog recovery • Rest of run easy	Rest
3	Step back	Strength training • Priority 4 • 5/10 effort Easy run • Priority 4 • 3 miles (4.8km) • Zone 2	Easy run with strides • Priority 3 • 4 miles (6.4km) • Warm up 15 mins, zone 2 • 4×60m strides with 60m jog recovery • Rest of run easy	Rest
4		Strength training • Priority 4 • 8/10 effort Easy run • Priority 4 • 6 miles (9.6km) • Zone 2	Easy run with strides • Priority 3 • 8 miles (12.9km) • Warm up 15 mins, zone 2 • 6×60m strides with 60m jog recovery • Rest of run easy	Rest
5		Strength training • Priority 4 • 8/10 effort Easy run • Priority 4 • 6 miles (9.6km) • Zone 2	Easy run with strides • Priority 3 • 9 miles (14.5km) • Warm up 15 mins, zone 2 • 8×60m strides with 60m jog recovery • Rest of run easy	Rest

Day 4	Day 5	Day 6	Day 7
Fartlek • Priority 2 • 6 miles (9.6km) • Warm up 15 mins, zone 2 • 4×60m strides with 60m jog recovery • 7×1 min at mixed pace from 5km to marathon with 1 min recovery • Rest of run easy	Strength training/cross train • Priority 5 • 8/10 effort • Zone 1–2 for 30 mins	Long run • Priority 1 • 13 miles (20.9km) • Zone 2	Rest
Steady run • Priority 2 • 6 miles (9.6km) • Zone 3	Strength training/cross train • Priority 5 • 5/10 effort • Zone 1–2 for 30 mins	Long run • Priority 1 • 8 miles (12.9km) • Zone 2	Rest
Fartlek • Priority 2 • 6 miles (9.6km) • Warm up 15 mins, zone 2 • 4×60m strides with 60m jog recovery • 6×1.5 min at mixed pace from 5km to marathon with 1.5 min recovery • Rest of run easy	Strength training/cross train • Priority 5 • 8/10 effort • Zone 1–2 for 30 mins	Long run • Priority 1 • 13 miles (20.9km) • Zone 2	Rest
Fartlek • Priority 2 • 6 miles (9.6km) • Warm up 15 mins, zone 2 • 4×60m strides with 60m jog recovery • 5×2 mins at mixed pace from 5km to marathon with 2 min recovery • Rest of run easy	Strength training/cross train • Priority 5 • 8/10 effort • Zone 1–2 for 30 mins	Long run • Priority 1 • 14 miles (22.5km) • Zone 2	Rest

Week	Focus	Day 1	Day 2	Day 3
6	Step back	Strength training • Priority 4 • 5/10 effort Easy run • Priority 4 • 3 miles (4.8km) • Zone 2	Easy run with strides • Priority 3 • 5 miles (8km) • Warm up 15 mins, zone 2 • 4×60m strides with 60m jog recovery • Rest of run easy	Rest
7		Strength training • Priority 4 • 8/10 effort Easy run • Priority 4 • 6 miles (9.6km) • Zone 2	Easy run with strides • Priority 3 • 10 miles (16km) • Warm up 15 mins, zone 2 • 8×60m strides with 60m jog recovery • Rest of run easy	Rest
8		Strength training • Priority 4 • 8/10 effort Easy run • Priority 4 • 6 miles (9.6km) • Zone 2	Easy run with strides • Priority 3 • 10 miles (16km) • Warm up 15 mins, zone 2 • 10×60m strides with 60m jog recovery • Rest of run easy	Rest
9	Step back	Strength training • Priority 4 • 5/10 effort Easy run • Priority 4 • 3 miles (4.8km) • Zone 2	Hill sprints • Priority 3 • 6 miles (9.6km) • Warm up 15 mins, zone 2 • 4×60m strides with 60m jog recovery • 6×30 secs hard uphill and walk back down • Rest of run easy	Rest

Day 4	Day 5	Day 6	Day 7
Steady run • Priority 2 • 6 miles (9.6km) • Zone 3	Strength training/cross train • Priority 5 • 5/10 effort • Zone 1–2 for 30 mins	Long run • Priority 1 • 9 miles (14.5km) • Zone 2	Rest
Fartlek • Priority 2 • 6 miles (9.6km) • Warm up 15 mins, zone 2 • 4×60m strides with 60m jog recovery • 3×5 mins at mixed pace from 10-mile to half marathon with 2 min recovery • Rest of run easy	Strength training/cross train • Priority 5 • 8/10 effort • Zone 1–2 for 30 mins	Long run • Priority 1 • 14 miles (22.5km) • Zone 2	Rest
Fartlek • Priority 2 • 6 miles (9.6km) • Warm up 15 mins, zone 2 • 4×60m strides with 60m jog recovery • 3×8 mins at mixed pace from 10-mile to half marathon with 3 min recovery • Rest of run easy	Strength training/cross train • Priority 5 • 8/10 effort • Zone 1–2 for 30 mins	Long run • Priority 1 • 15 miles (24.1km) • Zone 2	Rest
Steady run • Priority 2 • 6 miles (9.6km) • Zone 3	Strength training/cross train • Priority 5 • 5/10 effort • Zone 1–2 for 30 mins	Long run • Priority 1 • 10 miles (16km) • Zone 2	Rest

Week	Focus	Day 1	Day 2	Day 3
10		Strength training • Priority 4 • 8/10 effort Easy run • Priority 4 • 6 miles (9.6km) • Zone 2	Hill sprints • Priority 3 • 10 miles (16km) • Warm up 15 mins, zone 2 • 4×60m strides with 60m jog recovery • 6×30 secs hard uphill and walk back down • Rest of run easy	Rest
11		Strength training • Priority 4 • 8/10 effort Easy run • Priority 4 • 6 miles (9.6km) • Zone 2	Hill sprints • Priority 3 • 10 miles (16km) • Warm up 15 mins, zone 2 • 4×60m strides with 60m jog recovery • 6×30 secs hard uphill and walk back down • Rest of run easy	Rest
12	Step back	Strength training • Priority 4 • 5/10 effort Easy run • Priority 4 • 3 miles (4.8km) • Zone 2	Hill repeats • Priority 2 • 6 miles (9.6km) • Warm up 15 mins, zone 2 • 4×60m strides with 60m jog recovery • 400m easy, 400m hard uphill, 400m easy, 400m hard downhill (three sets) • Rest of run easy	Rest
13		Strength training • Priority 4 • 8/10 effort Easy run • Priority 4 • 6 miles (9.6km) • Zone 2	Easy run with intervals • Priority 3 • 10 miles (16km) • Warm up 15 mins, zone 2 • 6×30 secs at 5km effort with 30 secs jog recovery • Rest of run easy	Rest

Day 4	Day 5	Day 6	Day 7
Hill repeats • Priority 2 • 6 miles (9.6km) • Warm up 15 mins, zone 2 • 4×60m strides with 60m jog recovery • 400m easy, 400m hard uphill, 400m easy, 400m hard downhill (1 set) • Rest of run easy	Strength training/cross train • Priority 5 • 8/10 effort • Zone 1–2 for 30 mins	Long run • Priority 1 • 16 miles (25.7km) • Zone 2	Rest
Hill repeats • Priority 2 • 7 miles (11.2km) • Warm up 15 mins, zone 2 • 4×60m strides with 60m jog recovery • 400m easy, 400m hard uphill, 400m easy, 400m hard downhill (two sets) • Rest of run easy	Strength training/cross train • Priority 5 • 8/10 effort • Zone 1–2 for 30 mins	Long run • Priority 1 • 17 miles (27.3km) • Zone 2	Rest
Easy run with strides • Priority 3 • 6 miles (9.6km) • Warm up 15 mins, zone 2 • 8×60m strides with 60m jog recovery • Rest of run easy	Strength training/cross train • Priority 5 • 5/10 effort • Zone 1–2 for 30 mins	Long run • Priority 1 • 13 miles (20.9km) • Zone 2	Rest
Intervals • Priority 2 • 7 miles (11.2km) • Warm up 2 miles, zone 2 • 6×60m strides with 60m jog recovery • 5–7×2 mins at 5km effort with 2 min jog recovery • Rest of run easy	Strength training/cross train • Priority 5 • 8/10 effort • Zone 1–2 for 30 mins	Long run • Priority 1 • 18 miles (29km) • Zone 2 with last 8 miles at marathon pace	Rest

Week	Focus	Day 1	Day 2	Day 3
14		Strength training • Priority 4 • 8/10 effort Easy run • Priority 4 • 6 miles (9.6km) • Zone 2	Easy run with intervals • Priority 3 • 10 miles (16km) • Warm up 15 mins, zone 2 • 6×30 secs at 5km effort with 30 secs jog recovery • Rest of run easy	Rest
15	Step back	Strength training • Priority 4 • 5/10 effort Easy run • Priority 4 • 3 miles (4.8km) • Zone 2	Easy run with strides and race pace • Priority 2 • 5 miles (8km) • Warm up 15 mins, zone 2 • 6×60m strides with 60m jog recovery • 2 miles at half marathon pace • Rest of run easy	Rest
16		Strength training • Priority 4 • 3/10 effort Easy run • Priority 4 • 6 miles (9.6km) • Zone 2	Easy run with intervals • Priority 3 • 10 miles (16km) • Warm up 15 mins, zone 2 • 6×30 secs at 5km effort with 30 secs jog recovery • Rest of run easy	Rest
17		Strength training • Priority 4 • 8/10 effort Easy run • Priority 4 • 6 miles (9.6km) • Zone 2	Easy run with intervals • Priority 3 • 10 miles (16km) • Warm up 15 mins, zone 2 • 6×30 secs at 5km effort with 30 secs jog recovery • Rest of run easy	Rest

Day 4	Day 5	Day 6	Day 7
Intervals • Priority 2 • 7 miles (11.2km) • Warm up 2 miles, zone 2 • 6×60m strides with 60m jog recovery • 3–4×4 mins at 5km effort with 4 min jog recovery • Rest of run easy	Strength training/cross train • Priority 5 • 8/10 effort • Zone 1–2 for 30 mins	Long run • Priority 1 • 19 miles (30.5km) • Zone 2	Rest
Mobility training • Priority 5 • 3/10 effort	Easy run with strides • Priority 3 • 2 miles (3.2km) • Warm up 15 mins, zone 2 • 6×60m strides with 60m jog recovery • Rest of run easy	Half marathon race • Priority 1 • 13.1 miles (21.1km)	Rest
Intervals • Priority 2 • 7 miles (11.2km) • Warm up 2 miles, zone 2 • 6×60m strides with 60m jog recovery • 2–3×6 mins at 5km effort with 6 min jog recovery • Rest of run easy	Strength training/cross train • Priority 5 • 8/10 effort • Zone 1–2 for 30 mins	Long run • Priority 1 • 20 miles (32.2km) • Zone 2	Rest
Intervals • Priority 2 • 8 miles (12.9km) • Warm up 2 miles, zone 2 • 6×60m strides with 60m jog recovery • 3–4×800m at 5km effort with 5 min jog recovery • Rest of run easy	Strength training/cross train • Priority 5 • 8/10 effort • Zone 1–2 for 30 mins	Long run • Priority 1 • 20 miles (32.2km) • Zone 2 with last 10 miles at marathon pace	Rest

Week	Focus	Day 1	Day 2	Day 3
18	Taper	Strength training • Priority 4 • 5/10 effort Easy run • Priority 4 • 3 miles (4.8km) • Zone 2	Intervals • Priority 2 • 7 miles (11.2km) • Warm up 2 miles, zone 2 • 6×60m strides with 60m jog recovery • 4–6×4mins at 5km effort with 4 min jog recovery • Rest of run easy	Rest
19	Taper	Strength training • Priority 4 • 5/10 effort Easy run • Priority 4 • 3 miles (4.8km) • Zone 2	Time trial • Priority 2 • 8 miles (12.9km) at marathon pace	Rest
20	Race week	Mobility training • Priority 4 • 3/10 effort	Easy run with strides • Priority 2 • 6 miles (9.6km) • Warm up 2 miles, zone 2 • 6×60m strides with 60m jog recovery • 2 miles at goal race pace • Rest of run easy	Rest

Day 4	Day 5	Day 6	Day 7
Easy run with strides • Priority 3 • 6 miles (9.6km) • Warm up 15 mins, zone 2 • 6×60m strides with 60m jog recovery • Rest of run easy	Strength training/cross train • Priority 5 • 5/10 effort • Zone 1–2 for 30 mins	Long run • Priority 1 • 15 miles (24.1km) • Zone 2	Rest
Easy run with strides • Priority 3 • 4 miles (6.4km) • Warm up 15 mins, zone 2 • 6×60m strides with 60m jog recovery • Rest of run easy	Strength training • Priority 5 • 5/10 effort	Long run • Priority 1 • 10 miles (16km) • Zone 2	Rest
Rest	Easy run with strides • Priority 3 • 2 miles (3.2km) • Warm up 15 mins, zone 2 • 6×60m strides with 60m jog recovery • Rest of run easy	Marathon race • Priority 1 • 26.2 miles (42.2km) • Race pace	Rest

CHAPTER 19

Strength

Strength is much more than just being able to pick up something heavy. I believe it means being both physically and mentally strong. The two go hand in hand and the process of gaining physical strength grows mental strength.

We need to be strong to:

- Carry out daily living tasks – this is called functional strength.
- Counteract age-related changes that will work against our strength in the future.
- Run well and be injury free.
- Cope mentally with the challenges of menopause, running and life.

We have learned that muscle mass naturally declines with age (see chapter 11). If we do nothing, we will get weaker. We need to take action to maintain and build muscle, and ignore the limits that others are so keen to put on us.

When it comes to running, strength is not just about lifting heavy weights. Agility, coordination and explosiveness of movements are crucial, too. Both low- and high-impact activities build strength. Heavy weights have their place, but first we need to learn how to move our body well, with good form and control. The basics of good nutrition, incremental training and recovery are also essential for strength-building.

> 'This is the one thing that I feel might be improving. I can't run as fast or do the bouncy stuff in gym classes as well, but I can increase the weights and feel like I'm having a decent workout. It definitely helps keep injuries at bay.'
> **Anonymous**

I've enlisted the help of personal trainer and runner Clare Clark for the remainder of this chapter. This is a book about running and menopause, not about weight lifting and menopause. As runners, there are differences in the approach we should take to strength training. Clare completely understands this and has created a selection of workouts to give you all-round body strength that will serve you in daily life and in your running.

Meet the expert: Clare Clark

Clare Clark is the owner and founder of Highfivefitness, a private gym in Newcastle. She is a qualified personal trainer and strength and conditioning coach and strongly believes that exercise should be accessible to all, without limitation. A keen runner, Clare has completed events of all distances, and built up her running and physical strength through many variants of exercise, such as strength and flexibility. It was this adaptability to exercise that made her realise the true importance of health, both physically and mentally. Clare shares her passion for running and strength with clients, helping them get ready for race day, improve PBs or simply get out of the door. Her philosophy is that exercise is not just about physical strength, it's about building friendships and communities, improving mental health, and building self-respect and confidence.

Website: highfivefitness.co.uk, Instagram: @highfivefitnessuk

CLARE'S THOUGHTS ON STRENGTH

Studies have shown that if you're able to exercise, then you can increase your muscle mass, strength and mobility, regardless of what stage of menopause you are at. There are many benefits to strength training, including:

- Increased leg strength.
- Increased bone density.
- Increased muscle mass.
- Improved pelvic floor strength.
- Reduced risk of injuries.

- Improved metabolic responses, for example heart rate and blood pressure, and reducing menopause symptoms, such as hot flushes.

There are many forms of strength training and this can feel overwhelming, especially if you're new to it. We're going to focus on strength training that's beneficial for your general health, but also your running performance. We'll focus on strengthening the individual muscles that we use when we're running, as well as building overall strength and endurance.

Barriers to strength training

Certain issues come up repeatedly with the women that I train. Runners are generally reluctant to swap a run for a strength session. It may feel counterproductive when in fact it can be the absolute opposite. Increasing your strength training can improve your running performance. It not only builds physical strength, but also mental resilience and confidence.

Many of my clients start to experience injuries and niggles when they hit menopause, and this can make them doubt their body and its abilities. Personal training is not an option for everybody, but if you do have access, talk to your personal trainer about your menopause and any struggles or changes you're experiencing, so they can adapt your training to help support you.

A major barrier to strength exercise is just not knowing where to start. My advice is always to keep it simple. Concentrate on building up strength slowly and do focused training on the key muscles used in running, to replicate your running-movement patterns. Time is a barrier for most women, but don't view strength training as an additional pressure. Swapping a run for a strength session will reap rewards. If getting to a gym is out of the question, there are plenty of things you can do at home. To help you, I've designed three home or gym strength programmes which focus on full-body strength, plyometrics and core, specifically for runners.

GOOD TO KNOW

Yoga and pilates can be extremely beneficial to runners and can be incorporated into a training programme. They are both low-impact workouts with a focus on strength and flexibility. Running is a high-impact activity, so it's ideal to have low-impact options alongside it, especially when menopause symptoms make high-impact activity impossible. Gaining core strength and flexibility improves both form and running efficiency. Pilates and yoga also train breath work and learning to synchronise breath work with movement can have a beneficial effect when translated into running. Yoga, in particular, trains balance and strength. Running requires good balance due to the single-leg nature of the sport and improving balance is key for injury prevention and running performance. I recommend including yoga and pilates practices in conjunction with the functional strength-based training in this book.

'I've started strength training to allow me to carry on playing hockey. I hate the gym, but I really don't wish to stop playing, especially since there is something that can be done. Finding the right gym is the most important thing.'
Nikki Carpenter

FUNCTIONAL STRENGTH TRAINING

When training my running clients, I adopt a functional training approach which means focusing the strength training on everyday movements and creating exercises that mimic these, for example a squat mirrors an everyday sit-to-stand movement. We then connect these everyday functional movements and develop them alongside the specific patterns that we use during running.

There are four main areas which running-specific strength training should incorporate and these are as follows:

- **Unilateral work**: Exercises that use one side of the body at a time help build strength in individual muscles and correct any imbalances. Running is effectively a single-leg activity and we rely on our single-leg strength. It's crucial to include unilateral training in all our running workouts.
- **Core**: This is essential for runners as a strong core helps running efficiency, which in turn improves endurance. Running is reliant on a strong core to help stabilise our hips and torso, which in turn provide us with a good running form. Core workouts also help to strengthen the pelvic floor muscles.
- **Plyometrics**: When we run, we can experience a force of up to three times our bodyweight. Plyometric training can replicate this force and strengthen our lower-body muscles to enable us to cope with this impact.
- **Balance and coordination**: Training balance and coordination is another essential. These will help you do the exercises themselves, improve your running and set you up for a healthy future (see chapter 18).

> 'I've definitely benefited from strength work. I haven't had many injuries and I'm sure it's due to lifting weights and doing single-leg strength exercises.'
> **Jodi Clouston-Kerr**

Choosing a weight

How do you choose the right weight of kettlebell (KB) or dumbbell (DB)? If you're new to strength training, it's sensible to start with a low weight, between 2 and 5 kilograms. You then need to ensure that you can perform repetitions (reps) with proper form. As your form improves, and if you feel that you're completing the reps with ease, it's time to increase the weight. As runners we want to build our strength and endurance, so aim to perform 10 to 15 reps of each exercise.

As a personal trainer, I use the rate of perceived exertion (RPE) test to establish whether a client is finding an exercise too difficult or too easy. This establishes how hard you are working on a scale of 1 to 10, with 1 being very easy and 10 being maximum effort. As a guide, if you're struggling to complete a set of 10 reps with good form and feel you're working at full effort (RPE 8 to 10) throughout the entire set, then decrease the weights so you can complete the full set more easily. In general, you should be aiming to complete a full set with good form, with hard effort (RPE 7 to 8) in the last couple of reps of the set. If you feel the intensity is low throughout the set, then increase your weights. If you aren't ready, or can't increase your weights, you can increase the number of reps instead, which will also raise the intensity of the workout. For example, start with 8 to 10 reps and once this feels comfortable, increase to 12 to 15 reps per exercise. Correct form is vital and it's better to use lighter weights or do fewer reps and maintain proper form throughout the full set.

'I'm doing more strengthening all the time, working heavier and harder rather than lots of reps at low weight. I'm finding it very effective in helping me feel good and strong, maintain my running form and minimise injuries.'
Claire Callaghan, Bristol

Timing your strength workouts

It's advisable to do a strength session either before a rest day or before an easy run day. Your muscles will be fatigued after strength training, so avoid doing intense running sessions the day after or the day before a strength workout to ensure that you get the full benefit.

As with running, the key is to build consistency with your strength training. When starting out, try to be patient and don't push too hard too soon. Focus on your form, allow yourself time to recover and, most importantly, enjoy it!

THE WORKOUTS

Aim to strength train twice a week. Each workout will take between 30 and 45 minutes, and make sure you warm up well before you begin. These three workouts include supersets. For example, in workout 1 there are four supersets called A, B, C and D. Perform each of these supersets three or four times before taking a short rest and moving on to the next one.

WORKOUT 1: STRENGTH

	Exercise	Equipment	Reps/sets
A1	Squat side walk	Resistance band	10 each direction
A2	Narrow squat to high knee	Resistance band	5 each leg
B1	Single-leg deadlift	KB/DB	5–10 each leg
B2	Single-arm row	KB/DB	10 reps each arm
C1	Reverse lunge	DB/KB	10 each leg
C2	Squat to high pull	DB/KB	10
D1	Kneel to push press	DB	10
D2	Single-leg glute bridge	Bodyweight	10 each leg

A1 Squat side walk

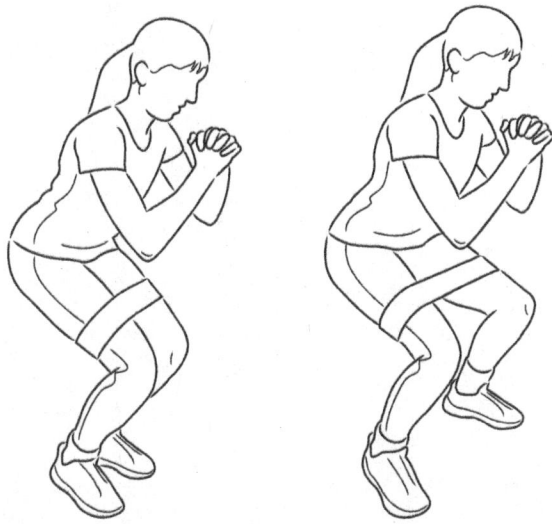

1. Place band just above your knees, around your thighs.
2. Bend your knees slightly. Maintain a squat position.
3. Take small sidesteps, keeping tension on the band.
4. Keep your hips level and knees bent. As you move, drive your knees directly over your midfoot, pushing outward against the band.

Progression
- Add a dumbbell, holding it to your chest in both hands.
- Increase resistance-band strength.
- Increase the depth of the squat.

Regression
Remove resistance band.

A2 Narrow squat to high knee

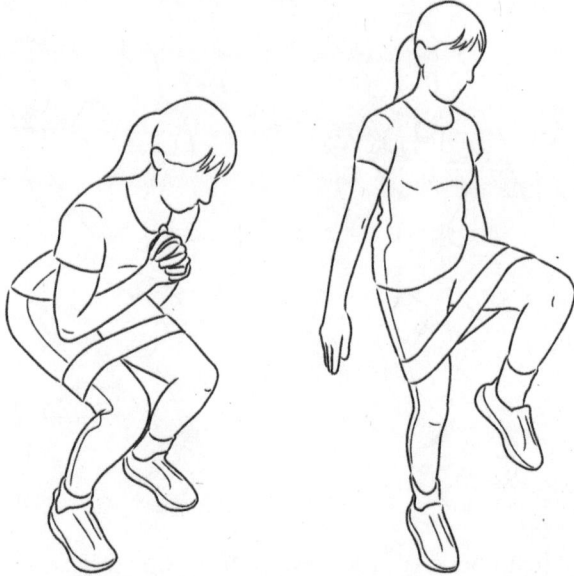

1. Place band just above your knees, around your thighs, with your feet hip-width apart and toes pointing forward.
2. Push your hips backwards and bend your knees as though sitting down in a chair. Aim for your hips to be below your knees on the down movement. Keep your chest lifted and shoulders back.
3. Stand up from squat position.
4. Drive your knee upwards towards your chest.
5. Repeat the movement, alternating the knee drive.

Progression
- Add dumbbells; hold one in each hand.
- Slow the downward tempo and increase the upward tempo.
- Increase the resistance-band strength.

Regression
Remove resistance band.

B1 Single-leg deadlift

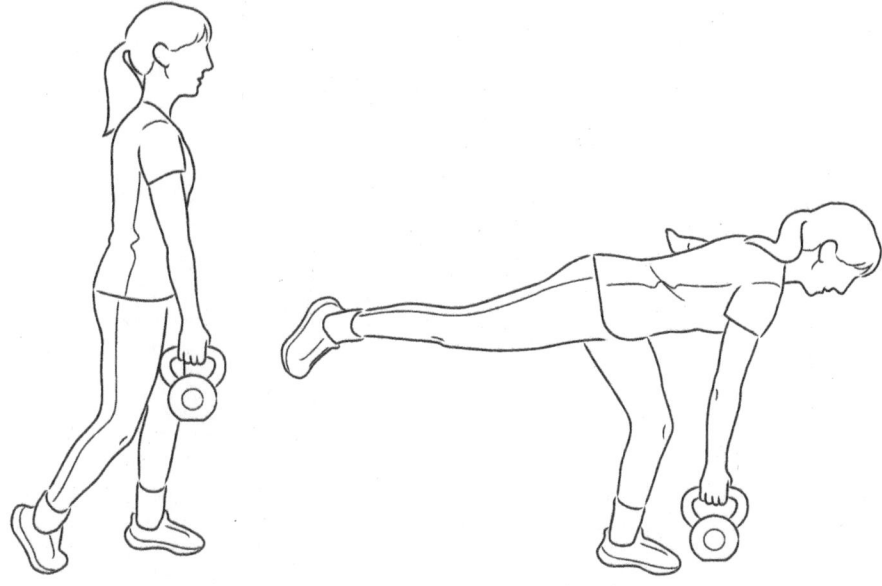

1. Lift one foot slightly off the floor and hold a balanced position. Maintain a soft knee in your standing leg. Hold a weight in the hand on the side of the moving leg.
2. Hinge at the hips and lean forward with your torso while lifting up your back leg.
3. Keep your back leg parallel with the torso and your head in neutral position, with your shoulders and hips square to the floor.
4. Return your foot to the floor while raising your torso back to the start position.

Progression
Add a knee drive at the top of the movement.

Regression
Use your bodyweight.

B2 Single-arm row

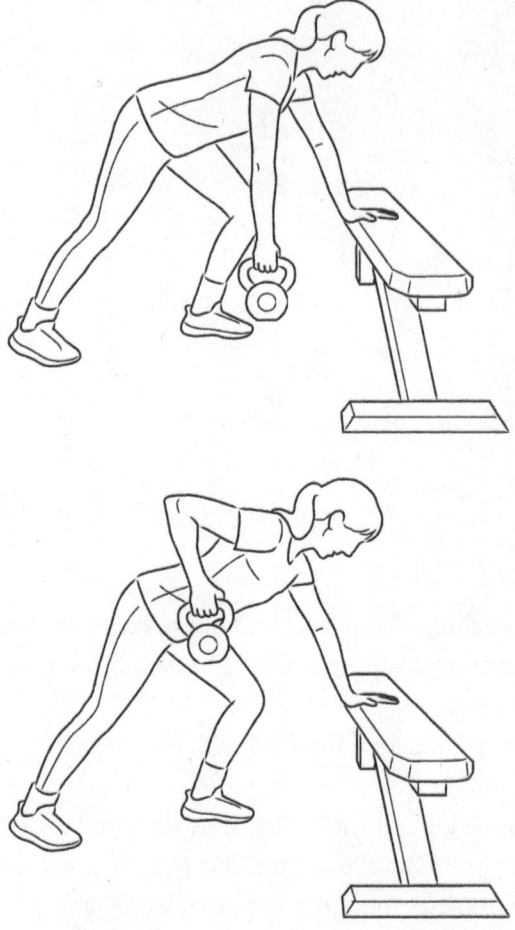

1. Place one leg forward and your resting arm on a bench or chair.
2. Engage your core, contracting your abdominal muscles to support your spine and maintain a straight back.
3. Keep your shoulders, head and spine in neutral position.
4. Exhale and pull the dumbbell upwards, bending your elbow towards your hip.
5. Squeeze your shoulders together at the top of the movement and keep your neutral back position.
6. Inhale, retract your shoulders and return the dumbbell to start position.

C1 Reverse lunge

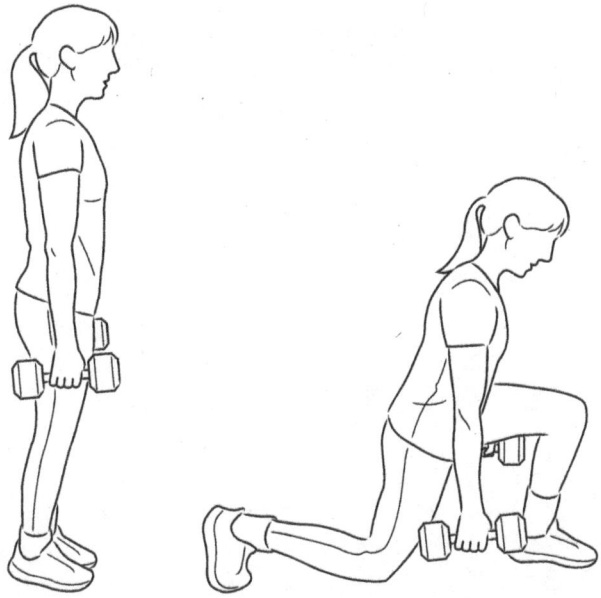

1. Start with your feet hip-width apart, holding dumbbells in both hands.
2. Step backwards, taking your knee straight down towards the floor.
3. Keep your front knee aligned with your second toe. Do not take your front knee over your toes.
4. Maintain neutral head and spine alignment.
5. Touch your back knee gently to the floor.
6. Engage your core muscles throughout and engage your glutes as your back leg returns to the start position.

Progression
- Add a resistance band around your thighs above your knees.
- Hold the dumbbells on your shoulders.

C2 Squat to high pull

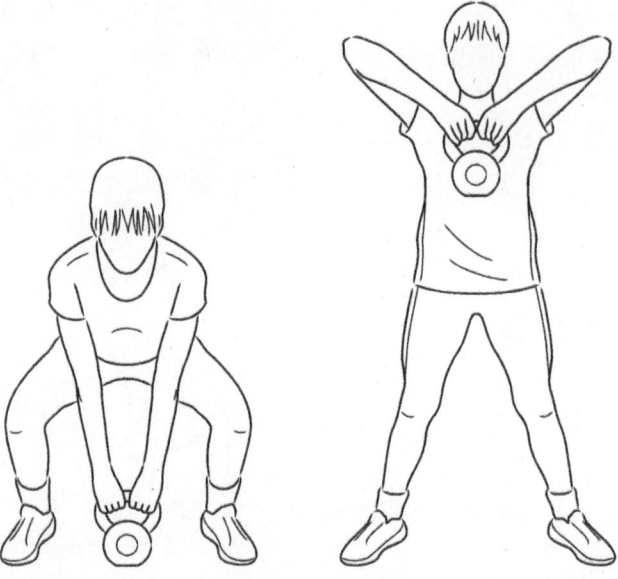

1. Stand with your feet wider than hip-width apart, toes slightly pointing outwards and holding a kettlebell in both hands.
2. Hinge at your hips, pushing backwards as though sitting down in a chair. Take the weight to the floor.
3. Maintain neutral spine straight back, and inhale.
4. Exhale, drive through your heels and power your legs vertically.
5. Once your legs are straight, drive your elbows up and out. Maintain a tight grip on the weight and keep it close to your chest.
6. Return to the start position.

Progression
- Slow the downward tempo of the movement.
- Increase the squat depth.

D1 Kneel to push press

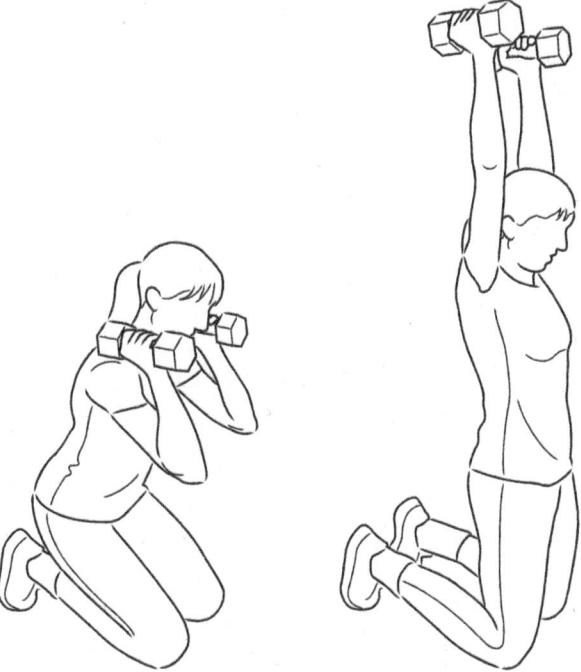

1. Kneel with both knees on the floor, hip-width apart. Place dumbbells on your shoulders.
2. Hinge at your hips, push your glutes over the heels and inhale.
3. Exhale and drive your hips forward, using your legs to create power.
4. Extend your hips and drive your arms upwards, pushing the weights to the ceiling.

Regression

If it is difficult to kneel, this exercise can be performed standing as a push press. Alternatively, a half-kneeling position can be used with one knee up and one knee down to add stability through the hips.

D2 Single-leg glute bridge

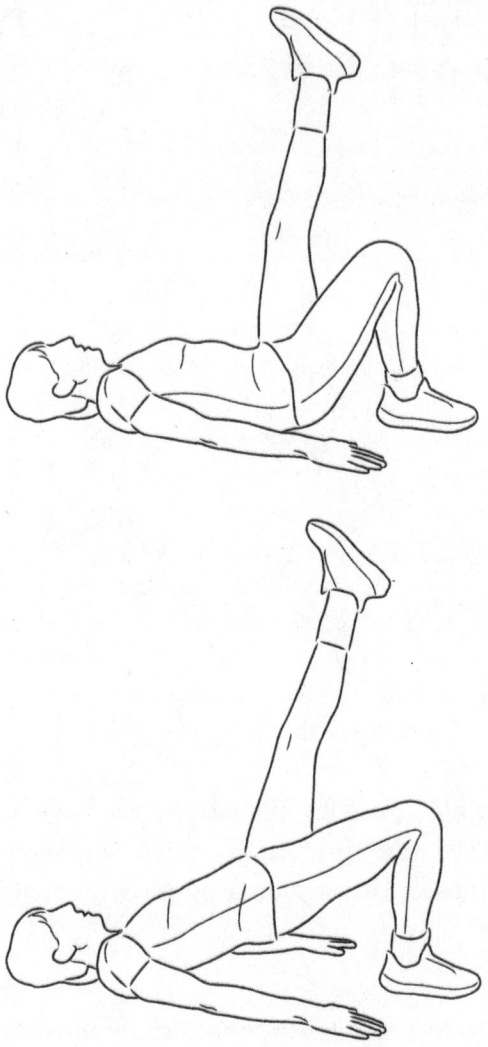

1. Lie on your back with your feet on the floor and knees hip-width apart.
2. Engage your core, pulling your belly button to your spine. Place your working leg firmly on the ground and raise the other leg.
3. Push through the working heel, lifting your hips off the floor, but ensuring they remain level and avoiding rotation.

4. Create a straight line from your shoulders to your working leg knee.
5. Squeeze your glutes at top of the movement and return to the start position.

Progression
- Hold a weight in both hands above your chest.
- Elevate your feet and place your working foot on a chair.

Regression
Keep both feet on the floor.

WORKOUT 2: BODYWEIGHT STRENGTH AND PLYOMETRICS

	Exercise	Reps
A1	Double pogo jumps	10–20
A2	Curtsy lunge to knee drive	5 reps each side
B1	Reverse lunge to knee drive	10 each leg
B2	Skater jumps	10 reps each side
C1	Squat jumps	10
C2	Single-leg sit to stand	5 reps each leg
D1	Burpees	10
D2	Double lateral hops	10 each side

A1 Double pogo jumps

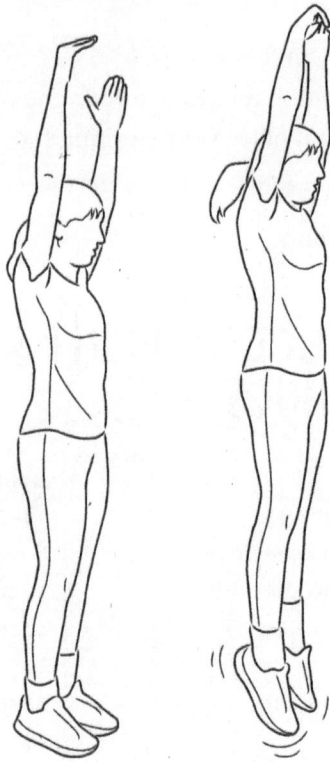

1. Maintain a slight knee bend throughout the movement, on landing and on the rebound.
2. Use your ankles and calves to power a vertical jump, taking your arms above the head.
3. Land on the ball of your foot and, on landing, spend minimal time on the floor before the rebound.
4. Keep your core engaged throughout the movement, holding a tall, upright position.
5. Repeat the bounce, fast and high like a pogo stick.

Progression
Single-leg pogo jumps.

Regression
Double calf raises without the jump.

A2 Curtsy lunge to knee drive

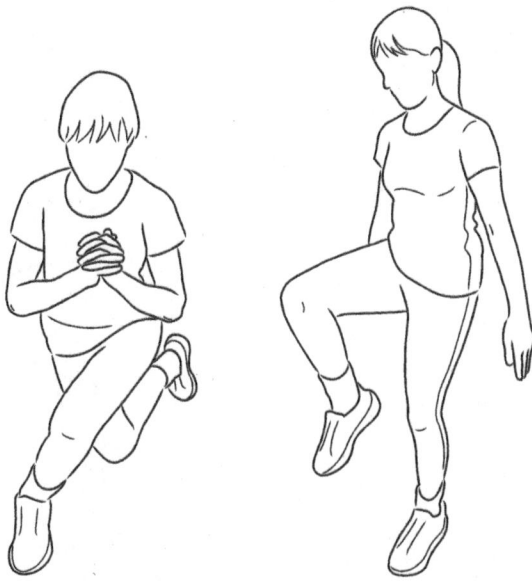

1. Start with your feet hip-width apart. Maintain a square hip position, keeping your hip bones pointing forwards.
2. Step diagonally back with one leg, so it crosses behind the stationary leg.
3. Bend both knees, taking your back knee towards the floor and keep your front knee aligned with your front ankle.
4. Engage your core throughout. Squeeze your glutes and drive your back leg to the top, stabilising through your stationary leg.
5. Drive the knee of your back leg up to balance at the top of the movement.
6. Place your elevated foot back on the floor.

Progression
- Add a pulse at the base of the movement.
- Do not place the moving foot on the floor between reps.

B1 Reverse lunge to knee drive

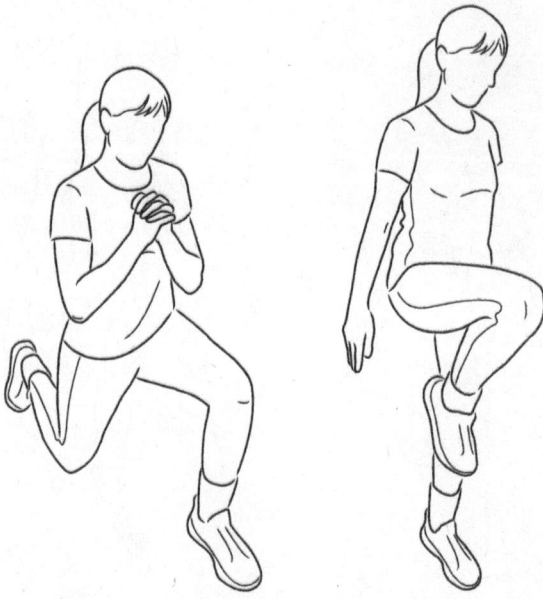

1. Take a long stride back and bend through both knees, taking your back knee towards the floor.
2. Engage your core, maintaining a straight posture with your shoulders back throughout the movement.
3. On return to standing raise your back leg and drive your knee towards your chest.
4. Drive the weight through your front foot to control the movement.
5. Pause at the top. Return your foot to the start position.

Progression
- Add a single-leg jump at the end of the movement with your standing leg.
- Do not place your moving foot on the floor between reps.

Regression
Remove the knee drive.

B2 Skater jumps

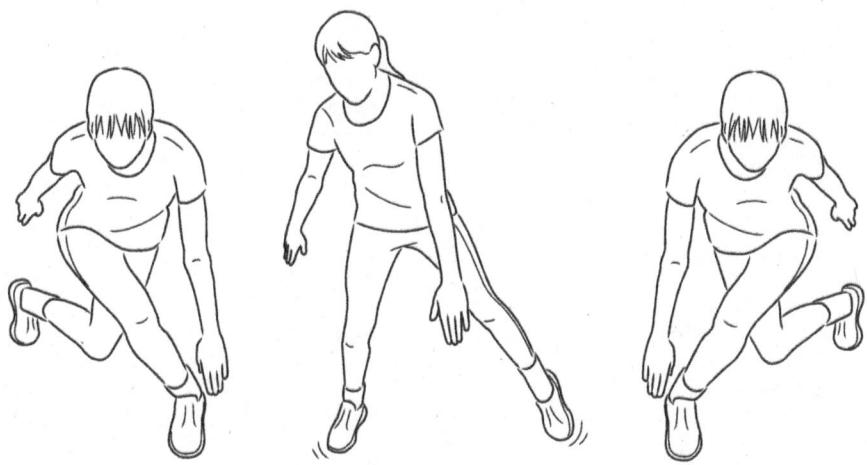

1. Start with your feet shoulder-width apart. Shift your weight to one leg, take your other leg behind your front leg, bend your knees and lower your hips.
2. Push off from your standing leg and jump laterally. Swing your arms across your body in the direction of the jump. Land gently on the opposite leg, crossing the other behind, bending both knees and lowering your hips.
3. Aim for an explosive movement. Engage your glutes and core to ensure control throughout.

Regression
To reduce impact, remove the jump. Step through the movement performing a curtsy. Do not place the trailing foot on the floor behind to work on building balance without the impact.

C1 Squat jumps

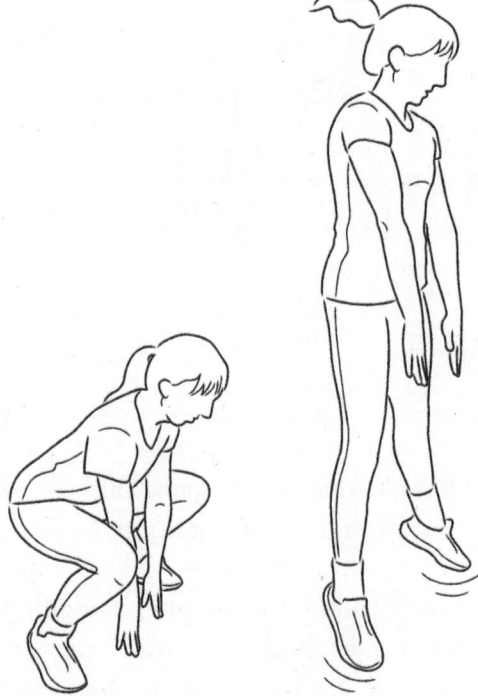

1. Stand with your feet wider than hip-width, toes pointing out.
2. Bend your knees, pushing your weight backwards over your heels. Lower your body and aim for your hips to be below your knees.
3. Explode upwards from the squat position. Maintain an engaged core throughout the movement, adding arm swings for power.
4. Bend your knees on landing to ensure the impact is absorbed. Return to the standing position.

Regression
Squat to calf raise.

C2 Single-leg sit to stand

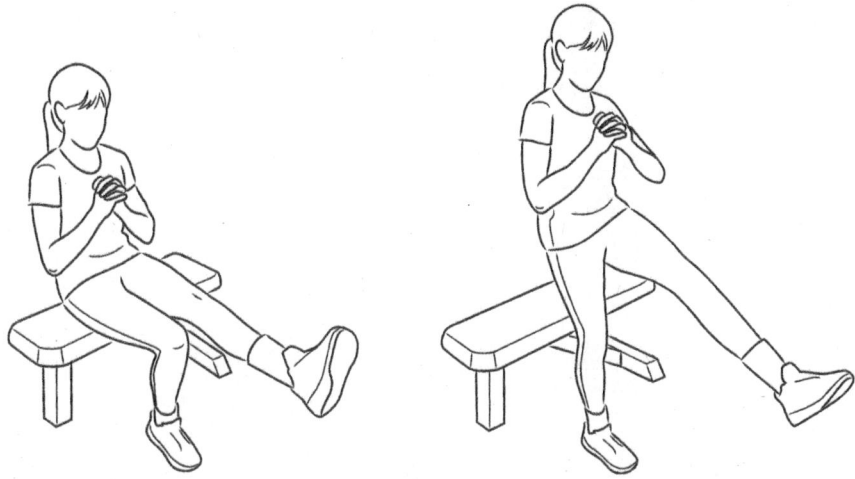

1. Sit on a chair which allows a 90-degree knee bend when seated.
2. Point one foot forwards. Clasp your hands to your chest or place them on your hips to avoid using your arms during the movement.
3. Lift the other foot off the floor and hold it up.
4. Push through the heel of your standing foot and straighten your knee.
5. Hold the single-leg stance at the top for balance.
6. Keep your leg lifted and slowly bend through the stationary leg. Return to the chair with a controlled descent.

Progression
- Slow the downward tempo of the movement.
- Remove the chair and increase your range of movement.

Regression
Place your feet in a staggered position, keeping both feet on the floor. Drive your weight through the foot closest to the chair.

D1 Burpees

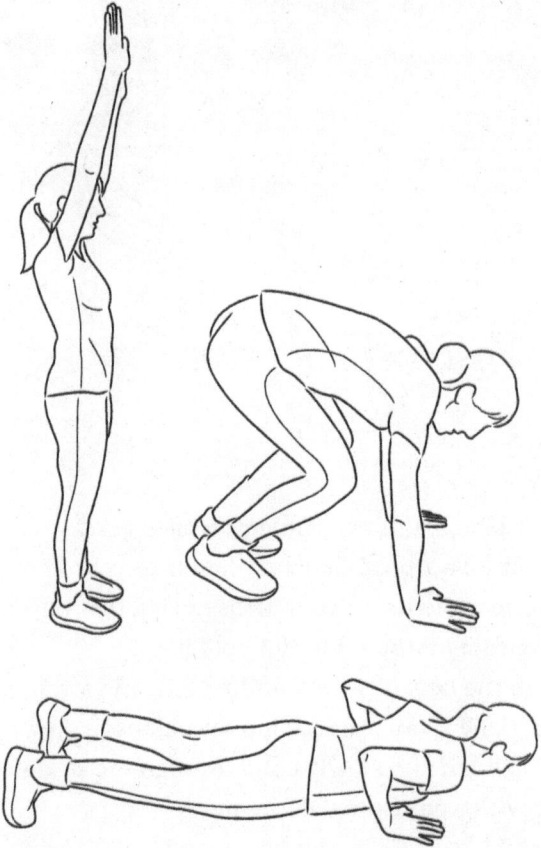

1. Start with your feet shoulder-width apart. Stand tall, eyes looking ahead.
2. Bend your knees. Place your hands on the floor and maintain a straight back.
3. Jump both feet back to a high plank position.
4. Bend your arms and take your chest to the floor.
5. Push your chest back up, jump your feet into your chest, sit back into a squat position and explode upwards to a vertical jump. Land softly with slightly bent knees.

Regression

Do a walkout burpee by placing your hands on the floor and stepping back one foot at a time to a plank position. Step your feet back to your hands and return to standing.

D2 Double lateral hops

1. Stand with your feet hip-width apart, knees slightly bent.
2. Push through the ground and jump both feet to the side. Keep your hips and knees bent and your torso vertical.
3. Land softly on the balls of your feet.
4. Immediately jump back to the other side.
5. Maintain a slight knee bend to absorb the impact.
6. Aim for a fast, explosive movement, adding arm swings for power.

Progression
Single-leg pogo jumps.

Regression
Step from side to side over an imaginary line. Once confident, add a small push off on the side-to-side movement.

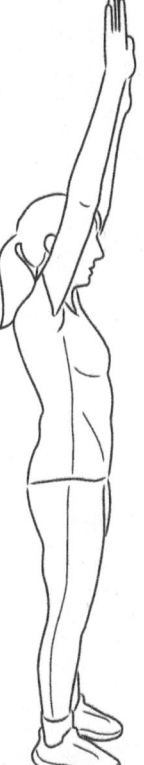

WORKOUT 3: CORE

	Exercise	Reps
A1	Inchworm	10
A2	Renegade row	5 each side
B1	Birddog	10 each side
B2	Mountain climbers	20
C1	Deadbug	10 each side
C2	Glute bridge	10
D1	Side plank leg raise	10 each side
D2	Plank	30 seconds

A1 Inchworm

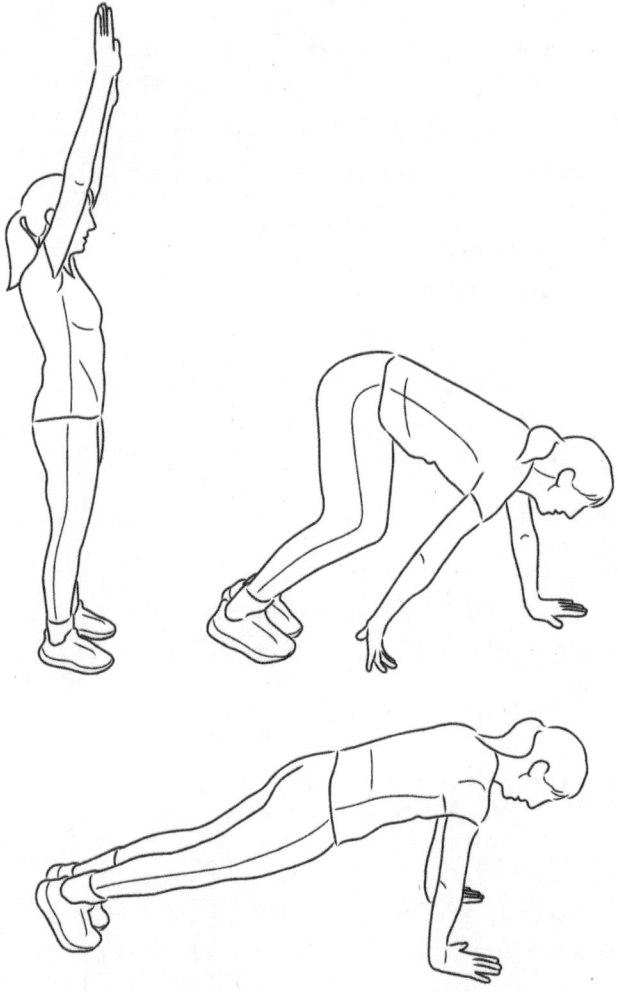

1. Start with your feet hip-width apart. Stand tall and engage your core. Raise your arms above your head.
2. Hinge at your hips, keep your back straight and place your hands towards the floor.
3. Walk your hands out, and reach the plank position, maintaining a straight line from head to heels. Squeeze your glutes and keep your core engaged to prevent your hips dropping.
4. Walk your hands back towards your feet, hinge at your hips and keep a straight back. Roll back up to a standing position.

A2 Renegade row

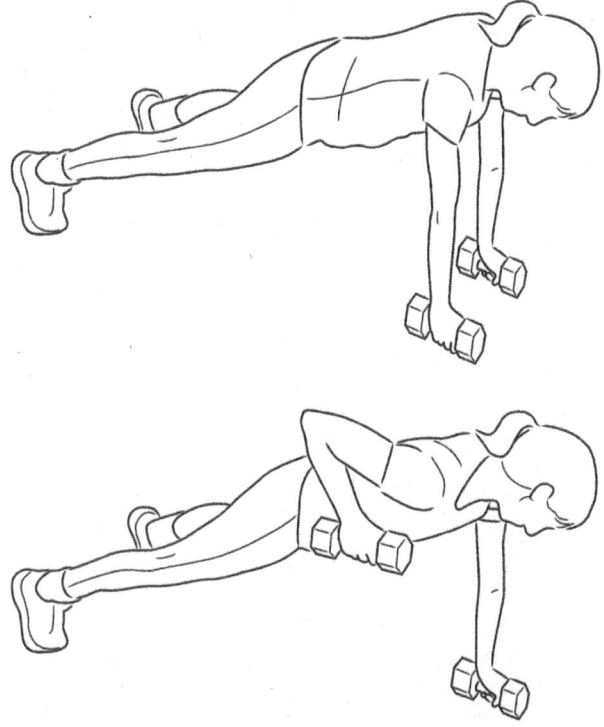

1. Start in a high plank position with a dumbbell in each hand and your hands directly under your shoulder.
2. Keep your feet hip-width apart and your glutes tight to maintain a straight line from head to heels.
3. Engage your core throughout the movement to avoid any rotation through your body.
4. Pull the dumbbell towards your chest, keeping your elbow tucked into your body.
5. Keep your hips pointing towards the floor to avoid rotation.
6. Squeeze your shoulder blades together during the movement.
7. Lower the dumbbell back to the floor at a controlled speed.

Regression

- Take your feet to a wider stance to ensure there is no rotation through your hips.
- Hold a half plank, keeping your knees on the floor.

B1 Birddog

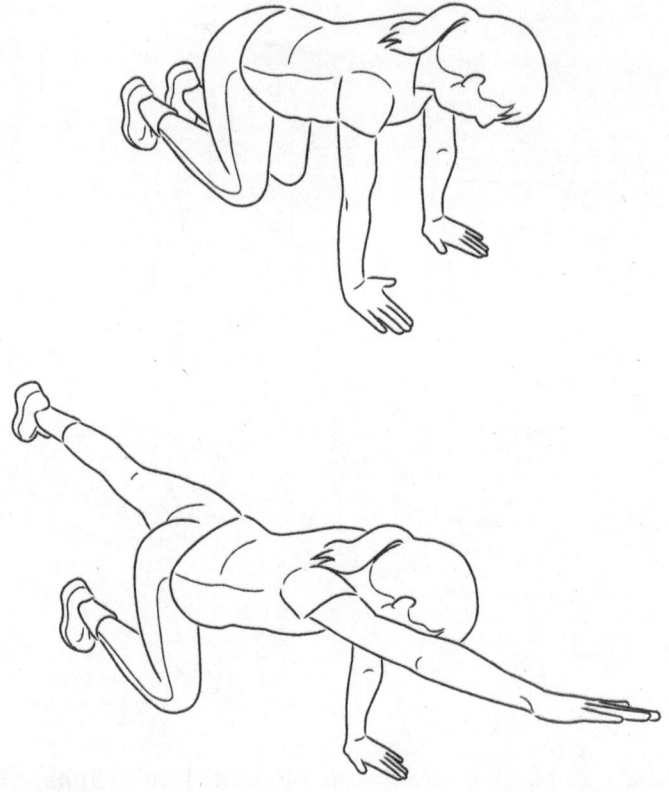

1. Start on all fours. Place your knees directly under your hips and your hands directly under your shoulders. Keep your back flat and ensure a straight line from the top of your head to your hips.
2. Engage your core by pulling your belly button towards your spine.
3. Extend your opposite arm and leg simultaneously. Create a straight line from your foot to your opposite hand.
4. Keep the movement slow and controlled, returning to the start position.
5. Keep your shoulders relaxed throughout and focus on not sagging through your back.

Regression

Move your opposite arm and then your opposite leg independently.

B2 Mountain climbers

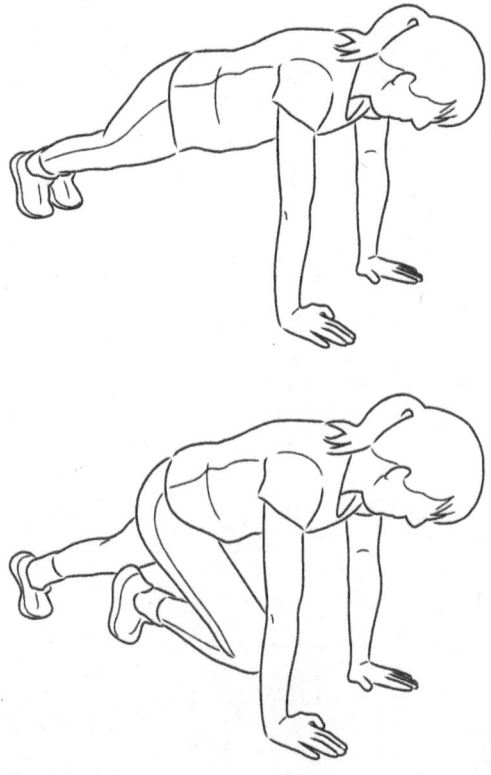

1. Start in a plank position. Engage your glute muscles and avoid dropping your hips.
2. Keep a straight line from the top of your head to your heels.
3. Inhale, then exhale and pull one knee towards your chest. Return your leg to the start position. Alternate between legs.
4. Keep control throughout the movement. Ensure your spine stays neutral and avoid lifting your hips.
5. Keep the movement slow and controlled, adding a pause at the top of the knee drive.

C1 Deadbugs

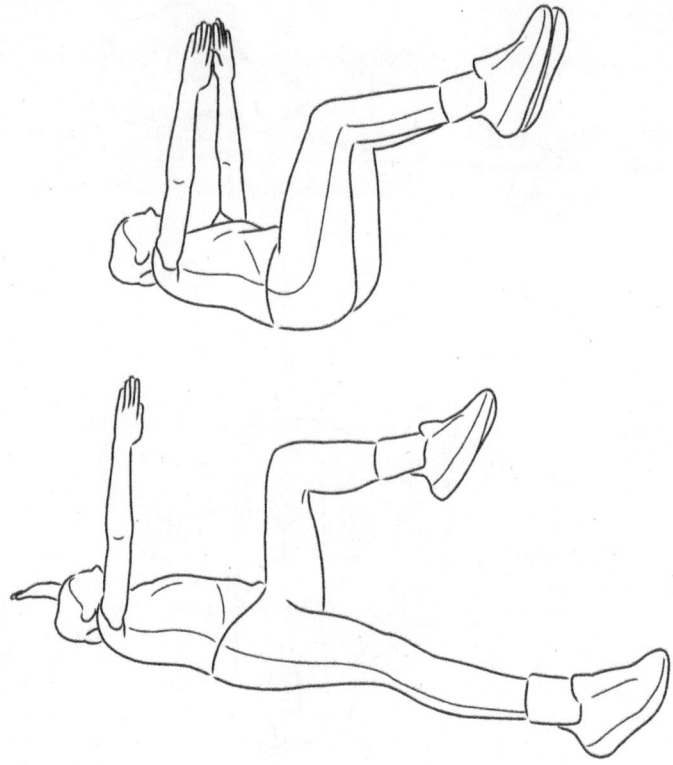

1. Lie on your back with your knees held at 90 degrees and your arms extended towards the ceiling.
2. Engage your core by drawing your belly button towards your spine.
3. Inhale, then exhale, and slowly and with control extend your opposite arm and leg out towards the floor.
4. Keep your core engaged throughout and avoid any arching in your lower back.
5. Return to the start position and repeat with your other arm and leg.

C2 Glute bridge

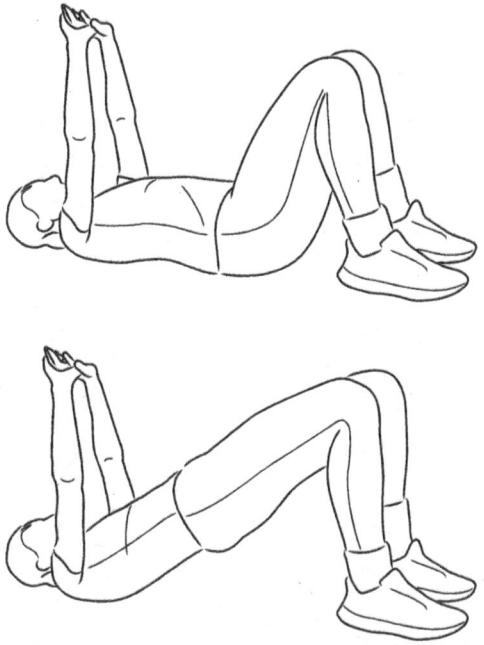

1. Lie on your back with your knees bent and feet hip-width apart, flat on the floor. Keep your heels directly under your knees.
2. Extend your arms towards the ceiling and hold them in that position.
3. Inhale, engage your core and squeeze your glutes.
4. Exhale, lift your hips off the floor, creating a straight line from your knees to your shoulders.
5. Maintain a neutral spine throughout.
6. Squeeze your glutes at the top of the movement. Slowly lower your hips and return to the start position.

Progression
- Place both feet on a chair for an elevated glute bridge.
- Raise one foot off the floor for a single-leg glute bridge.

D1 Side plank leg raise

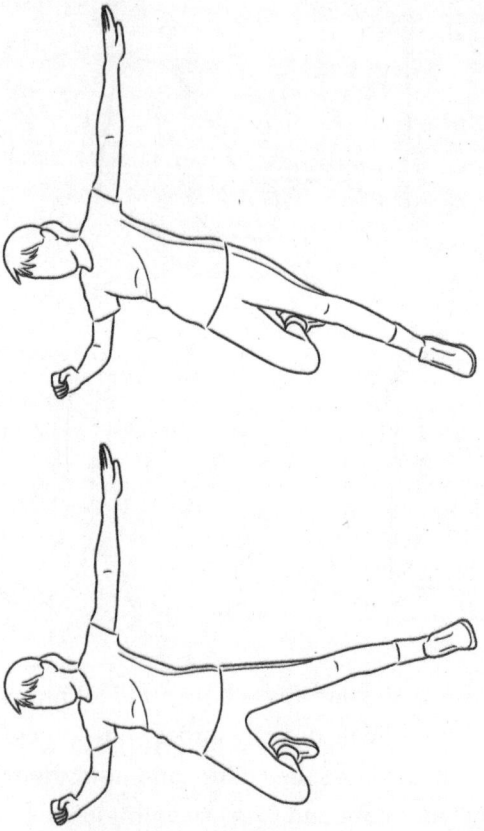

1. Lie on your side. Straighten your top leg and bend your bottom knee. Place your elbow directly under your shoulder.
2. Engage your core and squeeze your glutes, lifting your bottom hip.
3. Hold the side plank position and ensure your bottom hip doesn't dip.
4. Squeeze your glutes and raise your top leg up. Hold the movement at the top for two seconds and then return your foot to the floor in a slow and controlled manner.

Progression
Straighten your bottom leg for a full side plank.

Regression
Keep your bottom hip on the floor throughout the movement and just raise the top leg up and down.

D2 Plank

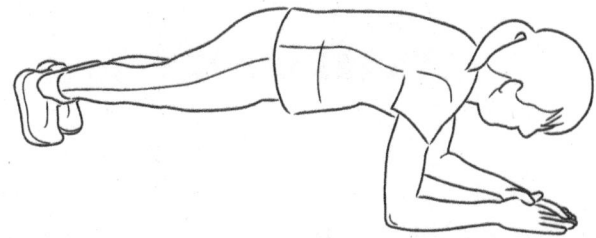

1. Place your elbows directly under your shoulders.
2. Keep your neck in alignment and look down to the floor.
3. Keep your shoulder blades down and pull away from the ears.
4. Keep your body in a straight line from head to heels.
5. Your back should be flat with the bottom down.
6. Squeeze your glutes throughout and imagine pushing the floor away from you.
7. Keep controlled breathing throughout.

Regression

Keep both knees on the floor for a half plank.

CHAPTER 20

Mindset

If you have days when you think you've got this whole menopause and running thing nailed and others when you feel you might as well hang up your trainers for good, then you are completely normal. In menopause, that kind of swing is absolutely to be expected. I've explained the effect that menopausal hormonal changes can have on your physical and mental abilities, so putting all the blame on yourself, and concluding that you're weak and can't cope, just isn't fair. It's not your fault. Yes, it's frustrating, annoying and even depressing, but beating yourself up and falling out of love with running is not going to help you. You need to keep running in your life for all the wonderful reasons we've discovered together. Give yourself a break and go at this with a positive mindset.

> 'I know a woman who says incredibly negative things about menopause. For example, "You'll put on weight and you'll never be able to shift it. Menopause sucks all the life and goodness out of us and leaves us with nothing." I've noticed a big difference in women depending on mindset. Women who are negative tend to not cope with it and don't help themselves to make sensible, positive changes, while those who are optimistic or more philosophical about it have an attitude of "When the going gets tough, the tough get going," and end up having great outcomes, and being fitter and more fantastic than ever. Whether you think you can or you think you can't, you're right. Ditch the negative mindset and don't project your toxic ideas onto other people.'
>
> **Anonymous**

MAKE THINGS EASY

I have a tendency to make things hard for myself – just ask my husband about the time we were on a multi-day hike and I chose not to have our rucksacks transported from place to place because I thought it would be more of a challenge to carry them over the gruelling hills ourselves. Big mistake! Menopause is not a time to be carrying any loads you don't need to. Look for the shortcuts, the easy options and the bag carriers. That also means not unnecessarily taking on other people's loads. Our growing wisdom can help us set clear boundaries and say, 'No'. You can't climb the mountain of menopause if you can hardly take a step forward from the weight of everyone else's burdens.

Avoid unnecessary pressure

Running must not become a pressure; there's enough on you already. Setting goals is a great way to stay motivated, but make sure they are realistic and achievable. Set yourself up for success and be patient with yourself. Accept that your running might change during this time and be open to running differently. Be curious on this journey of discovery and willing to try new things. Have a positive attitude, look at what you can change and control, and don't worry about the rest.

Keep the faith

Have belief in yourself that you can do this; that you are worth the extra time, energy and effort. Believe in your running and your future, powerful self. The science gives indisputable evidence that if you carry on being active, you will be healthier. Having others around you who believe in you is really important, especially if you struggle with self-belief, so find your cheerleaders in life. I believe in you.

'I joined a 261 club at a very low point and found that running didn't have to be competitive or pressured, which was the reason I stopped running when I was younger. Running can be fun, social, supportive and inclusive. Who knew?! This has been such a liberation, as has finally reaching menopause. These days I'm amazed and grateful for the strength in my body, and the confidence in general that my menopausal running has given me. We midlife women can do so much more than we imagine. Probably for the first time in my life I feel truly fearless!'

Helen L, Lancaster

Keep learning

There is always more to learn and I hope this book has increased your knowledge about what is happening in your body, so you feel more equipped to deal with all that is thrown at you. Learn as much as you can – from reputable sources. Educating yourself helps you feel capable and empowered. There will be a lot of trial and error, but learn from setbacks and find what works for you.

Consistency is key

Doing something daily is very powerful. Running every day isn't usually the best thing for most of us, but doing something, no matter how small, will keep us moving forwards. Consistent actions have huge rewards over time.

'I feel positive about menopause, and I'm keen to stay strong, active and keep running for as long as possible. I'm inspired by women I know who are still doing half marathons and marathons, and competitive shorter distances, in their sixties and seventies. It's also great to see Paula Radcliffe, who is my age, back doing distance running.'

Claire Callaghan, Bristol

MAKING CHANGES

Menopause gives us the ideal opportunity to make lifestyle changes and address how we live, what we eat and how we move. This is important whether we choose to use HRT or not. Making change is hard, but as I said in the introduction, it's been proven to be easier at times of life transition, so let's use menopause to our advantage.

When it comes to making changes, working out what really motivates you is important. This is a very personal thing and we all have different drivers. For me, it's the desire to be healthy and independent in my old age, so I can continue to enjoy my family and the outdoors. Even though I have that goal, it can still be difficult to go for that run! It's hard to be enthusiastic and motivated about much if you're in the throes of menopause, so we need to find another way.

We can't simply rely on our will power, because it runs out, especially towards the end of the day. So, what can we do? We can turn to discipline. Discipline is the ability to keep working at something that is difficult. By setting our own rules and keeping to them, we gain self-control. This in turn helps us feel confident in our ability to do hard things. This isn't about punishment, it's about making some things non-negotiable, so that we don't have to find motivation, use up will power or make a decision. It's just what we do, consistently, whether we're motivated or not.

This mindset shift has helped me enormously in menopause. I may not feel like doing a strength session, but it's just what I do when I get out of bed in the morning. There's no negotiation and it's a relief not to be having that internal dialogue. If I waited for the motivation, it would never happen. This is too important now. I know my future health depends on it and 80-year-old Juliet is cheering me on. After months of doing it, I'm seeing the benefits of that discipline, and strength work has become a habit. You can set great goals, you can plan rewards and be accountable, and this all helps, but at the end of the day, you still have to do the work. Discipline over motivation has worked for me and I hope it might help you, too.

'For much of my life, I was scared of menopause. I felt like it was the start of being old. I had problems with pain and heavy bleeding throughout my menstrual-cycle life, and knew the only chance I had of stopping it was to have it all ripped out. To be honest, for most of the first year after my hysterectomy I felt old. It wasn't until [marathon runner] Kathrine Switzer reminded me that I can do it that my mindset shifted. I laced up my trainers again and started to regain control over my life. I see this as my time now – my time to see what I am capable of.'

Lisa Ruggles, Oxford

HOW TO START

With a book like this, there's a risk of feeling that you just have a long list of to-dos and are too overwhelmed to know where to begin. You're ready to make change and tackle those menopausal running barriers, but where do you start? It can be even more of a challenge if everything is feeling hard and you can't see any positives. Having a process to work through can help. Here is mine:

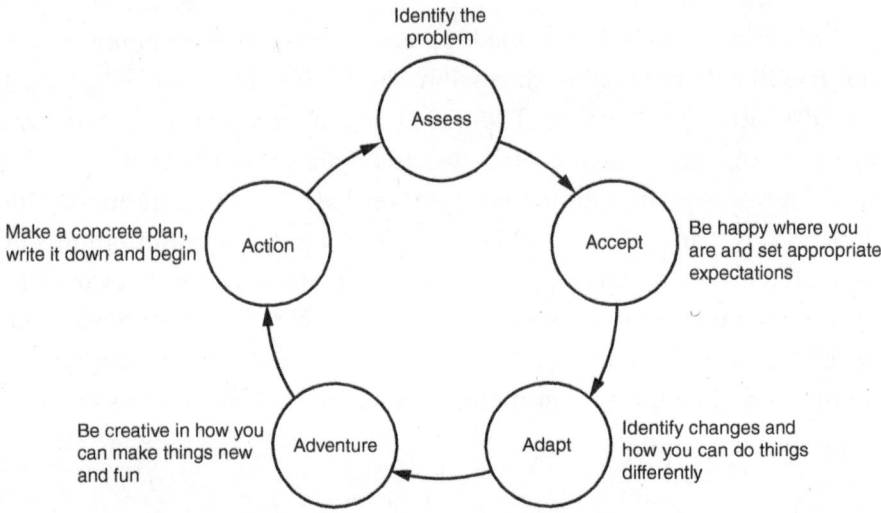

1. **Assess**: Work out exactly what's going on. Step back from the situation and imagine you're watching yourself. What is the issue that you're struggling with? What else is going on in life that might be affecting this? Maybe you're just being too hard on yourself? Don't forget, we all have bad-run days from time to time anyway, regardless of our hormonal status. Try to really identify the problems and what is influencing them.
2. **Accept**: This is the tricky one! It's easy to focus on what you feel you've lost. Instead, accept where you are now and adjust your expectations of yourself. That doesn't mean you can't make progress or push yourself, but meet yourself where you're at rather than focusing on where you think you should be. If you keep focusing on that gap, you'll always feel negative and overwhelmed. You are where you are meant to be right now. Accept that and make sure your expectations of yourself are appropriate.
3. **Adapt**: Think about what you can change to help the problem you've identified. Is there another way you can do things? When you've suffered a setback before, what did you learn and what helped you? Try to be open-minded and flexible here. Draw on what you've learned from this book to help you overcome the hurdles. Come up with some simple steps that you can take.
4. **Adventure**: How can you get yourself excited about implementing the steps? We can all be stuck in our ways. Sometimes we're just uncertain, afraid or lacking in confidence. Now is the perfect time to take a deep breath, add some adventure and try something new. You are wise and strong; you can do hard things. You don't have to do it on your own – ask a friend to help. It doesn't have to be a huge adventure. It's about finding the joy in small things and having some fun.
5. **Action**: Finally, you need to take action. Write your plan down. Make yourself accountable and share it with someone else if it will help you. Then get started. Don't overthink it, just begin, one day at a time.

Let's work through an example.

1. **Assess**: The problem is that I'm not motivated to run. Exploring this I realise it's because I'm getting slower, running is so hard and I'm not enjoying it. If I work it back, I see my reasons for getting slower are

because life has been busy and I haven't been running very consistently. When I do get out, I think I should be faster than I am. I'm disappointed and it puts me off running. Trying to run faster is hard. I'm so out of breath, which feels horrible. I'm not enjoying my runs, which doesn't help my motivation.

2. **Accept:** I need to be okay with the fact that running is feeling hard at the moment, which isn't unexpected in perimenopause. I've done well to keep going as long as I have. I can't expect to be running well if I'm hardly running. Beating myself up about being slow is just making me feel bad. I know there's more to running than speed and this isn't the beginning of the end. Running still has so much to offer me. I can accept where I am right now and I'm ready to take action.

Most people miss out this step and just jump on to making the plan, but don't do this. Take the time to really feel okay with where you are and think about how you will feel when you succeed.

3. **Adapt:** What could I change? I know that running consistently is key to me running well. I need to enjoy it more to be motivated to go. I don't have a lot of time and in the past I've learned that running more than three times a week isn't sustainable for me. Looking at my running stats is depressing me, so I could run without my watch. I really enjoy running with a friend, which helps to keep me accountable and motivated. I've learned that gaining muscle mass will help me increase my power and speed, so I could do a sprint interval session to help me build muscle and run faster.

4. **Adventure:** I'd love to explore some new, off-road routes. I won't do this on my own in case I get lost, but I could ask someone to join me. I've also learned that off-road running will be good for leg and core muscle strength, balance and coordination, so I'll be getting these benefits, too.

5. **Action:** My plan is to ditch my sports watch for a month. Once a week I'm going to do an off-road run with a friend with the aim of exploring, enjoying the scenery and chatting. I'm also going to do a sprint interval session once a week. I won't plan a third run, but I can add that later. I'll do this for four weeks. At that point I'll reward myself with a nice coffee with my running friend. I'll then reassess where I'm at and decide what's next.

I'm actually excited about the plan that I'm making, and feeling positive that I can get some joy and fun back into my running. I know if I make these changes I will feel more in control, more positive and like I'm doing something for myself. If I don't do anything I'm going to feel sluggish, and I can just see me running less and spiralling downwards, physically and mentally. Let's go!

Try this process out for yourself. Make sure you drill down to what the root of the problem is, keep working it backwards until you get there. Just focus on one or two things and be creative with your solutions. Adding some adventure will really help you with mindset, to find joy and do things differently. Go back to the relevant chapters to help you work out what action steps you can take. You can turn a problem into something positive by coming up with a plan that excites you and that you have control over. Fill your social media feeds with women who are thriving in post-menopause to remind you of that light at the end of the menopause tunnel.

'I keep going, because I love how running makes me feel like I can achieve anything.'
Jodi Clouston-Kerr

Closing Words

I hope this book has helped you realise that your best running days can still be ahead of you and the challenges of menopause will end. Whatever your level of running right now, it matters and is crucially important for your future. You need to make change, but you don't have to do it all at once. Success comes from being persistent and disciplined, and every tiny change you make counts and adds up over time.

I'm not pretending this is easy. Menopause can be an incredibly hard time of life. If running falls off your radar completely for a while, that's okay. Take a break, have a rest, do something else. Bring it back into your life when you're ready, in a gentle, pressure-free way. There are no rules here. That's the wonderful thing about running – it can be whatever you need it to be. It can flex and change, adapt and evolve. It doesn't mind if you ignore it for a bit, it's always willing to give you its power and magic, and will still be there for you. A life with running is a better life and a menopause with running is undoubtedly a better menopause. I hope I have helped you to keep running through yours. I believe you can and I hope you believe that yourself, too.

If you'd like to stay in touch, follow me on social media or subscribe to my weekly newsletter for menopausal runners. You can find all the links you need on my website: drjulietmcgrattan.com

Acknowledgements

I always get teary when I write this part of my books. Menopause has made me realise the power of women supporting women more than ever and when we work together we really can do incredible things.

Thank you to my publisher Charlotte Croft, editor Caroline Hewlett and the whole Bloomsbury team for giving me the opportunity to write about a topic that I'm passionate about, and for having me back for a third time!

A massive thank you to my experts whom I admire so much. Irene Clark, Dr Cath Munro, Renee McGregor, Clare Clark and Emma Brockwell – thank you for so generously sharing your time and expertise, and for all the amazing work you do to help women.

This book is so much richer for the words from women living through the journey of running in menopause. I'm so grateful to my newsletter readers, my 261 family and my coaching clients, who all shared their thoughts and experiences. It's you lot who inspire me to keep running and writing – thank you.

Finally, thank you to my friends and family, who stuck by me while I disappeared into my book-writing cave again. And to Horst, thank you for pushing me to challenge myself, learn more and become better, and for always trying to understand what it's like to be a woman.

References

Chapters 1–2

NICE guidelines [NG23]. (2015 – updated 2024) 'Menopause: identification and management'. nice.org.uk/guidance/ng23 [Accessed 2025].

British Menopause Society. (2021), 'What is the menopause?' thebms.org.uk/wp-content/uploads/2023/08/17-BMS-TfC-What-is-the-menopause-AUGUST2023-A.pdf [Accessed 2024].

British Menopause Society. (2023), 'Menopause in ethnic minority women'. thebms.org.uk/wp-content/uploads/2023/07/20-BMS-TfC-Menopause-in-ethnic-minority-women-JULY2023-B.pdf [Accessed 2024].

Davis, S.R., Taylor, S., Hemachandra, C., Magraith, K., Ebeling, P.R., Jane, F., Islam, R.M., (2023), 'The 2023 Practitioner's Toolkit for Managing Menopause'. Climacteric, 26(6), 517–536. doi.org/10.1080/13697137.2023.2258783.

El Khoudary, S.R., Greendale, G., Crawford, S.L., Avis, N.E., Brooks, M.M., Thurston, R.C., Karvonen-Gutierrez, C., Waetjen, L.E., Matthews, K. (2019), 'The menopause transition and women's health at midlife: a progress report from the Study of Women's Health Across the Nation (SWAN)'. Menopause. 26(10):1213–1227. doi.org/10.1097/GME.0000000000001424.

Tehrani, F.R., Solaymani-Dodaran, M.S., Hedayati, M., Azizi, F. (2010), 'Is polycystic ovary syndrome an exception for reproductive aging?' Human Reproduction, 25(7):1775–1781. doi.org/10.1093/humrep/deq088.

Bjelland, E.K., Hofvind, S., Byberh, L., Eskild, A., (2018), 'The relation of age at menarche with age at natural menopause: a population study of 336 788 women in Norway'. Human Reproduction, 33(6):1149–1157.

Chapter 3

Bansal, R., Aggarwal, N. (2019), 'Menopausal Hot Flashes: A Concise Review'. Journal of Midlife Health, 10(1): 6–13.

Huang, A., J., Grady, D., Jacoby, V.L., et al. (2008), 'Persistent Hot Flushes in Older Post-menopausal Women'. Archives of Internal Medicine, 168(8):840–846.

British Menopause Society. (2020 – updated 2023), 'Prescribable alternatives to HRT'. thebms.org.uk/wp-content/uploads/2022/12/02-BMS-TfC-Prescribable-alternatives-to-HRT-NOV2022-A.pdf [Accessed 2025].

British Menopause Society. (2022), 'Cognitive Behavioural Therapy (CBT) for Menopausal Symptoms'. thebms.org.uk/wp-content/uploads/2022/12/01-BMS-TfC-CBT-NOV2022-A.pdf [Accessed 2025].

Liu, T., Chen, S., Mielke, G.I., McCarthy, A.L., & Bailey, T.G. (2022), 'Effects of exercise on vasomotor symptoms in menopausal women: a systematic review and meta-analysis'. Climacteric, 25(6), 552–561. doi.org/10.1080/13697137.2022.2097865.

Bailey, T., Cable, N., Aziz, N., Atkinson, G., Cuthbertson, D Low, D., Jones, H. (2016), 'Exercise training reduces the acute physiological severity of post-menopausal hot flushes'. *Journal of Physiology* 594(3): 657–667.

Carpenter, J.S., Sheng, Y., Elomba, C.D., et al. (2021), 'A Systematic Review of Palpitations Prevalence by Menopausal Status'. *Current Obstetrics and Gynaecology Rep* 10, 7–13. doi.org/10.1007/s13669-020-00302-z.

Chapter 4

Salari, N., Hasheminezhad, R., Hosseinian-Farr, A., Rasoulpoor, S., Assefi, M., Nankali, S., Nankali, A., Mohammad, M. (2023), 'Global prevalence of sleep disorders during menopause: a meta-analysis'. *Sleep Breath,* Mar9:1-15. doi.org/10.1007/s11325-023-02793-5.

Bazeley, A., Marren, C., Shepherd, A. (2022), Fawcett Society. 'Menopause and the Workplace'. fawcettsociety.org.uk/menopauseandtheworkplace [Accessed 2024].

Patel, S.R., Malhotra, A., White, D.P., Gottlieb, D.J., Hu, F.B. (2006), 'Association between reduced sleep and weight gain in women'. *American Journal of Epidemiology,* 164(10):947–54. doi.org/10.1093/aje/kwj280.

Baker, F.C., Lampio, L., Saaresranta, T., Polo-Kantola, P. (2018), 'Sleep and sleep disorders in the menopausal transition'. *Sleep Medicine Clinics,* 13(3):443–456.

Kravitz, H.M., Joffee, H. (2011), 'Sleep During the Perimenopause: A SWAN Story'. *Obstetrics and Gynecology Clinics of North America,* 38(3):57–586.

Silvani, M.I., Werder, R., Perret, C. (2022), 'The influence of blue light on sleep, performance and wellbeing in young adults: A systematic review'. *Frontiers in Physiology,* 13:943108. doi.org/10.3389/fphys.2022.943108.

Lawrenson, J.G., Hull, C.C., Downie, L.E. (2017), 'The effect of blue-light blocking spectacle lenses on visual performance, macular health and the sleep-wake cycle: a systematic review of the literature'. *Opthalmic Physiol Opt,* 37:644–654. doi.org/10.1111/opo.12406.

Guthrie, K.A., Larson, J.C., Ensrud, K.E., Anderson, G.L., Carpenter, J.S., Freeman, E.W., Joffe, H., LaCroix, A.Z., Manson, J.E., Morin, C.M., Newton, K.M., Otte, J., Reed, S.D., McCurry, S.M. (2018), 'Nonpharmacologic Interventions on Insomnia Symptoms and Self-reported Sleep Quality in Women With Hot Flashes: A Pooled Analysis of Individual Participant Data From Four MsFLASH Trials'. *Sleep,* 41(1):zsx190. doi.org/10.1093/sleep/zsx190.

Kravits, H.M., Zhao, X., Bromberger, J.T., Gold, E.B., Hall, M.H., Matthews, K.A., Sowers M.R.R. (2008), 'Sleep Disturbance During the Menopause Transition in a Multi-Ethnic Community Sample of Women'. *Sleep,* 31(7):979–990.

Chapter 5

Cadegiani, F.A., Kater, C.E. (2016), 'Adrenal fatigue does not exist: a systematic review', *BMC Endocrine Disorders,* Aug;24;16(1):48. doi.org/10.1186/s12902-016-0128-4.

Endocrine Society. (2018), 'Adrenal Fatigue Debate', *Endocrine Society Podcast*, Dec 21, Episode 10 endocrine.org/podcast/enp10-adrenal-fatigue-debate [Accessed 2024].

Taylor-Swanson, L., Wong, A.E., Pincus, D., Butner, J.E., Hahn-Holbrook, J., Koithan, M., Wann, K., Woods, N.F. (2018), 'The dynamics of stress and fatigue across menopause: attractors, coupling and resilience'. *Menopause*, Apr;25(4):380–390.

NICE Guideline [NG206] (2021), 'Myalgic encephalomyelitis (or encephalopathy)/chronic fatigue syndrome: diagnosis and management'. nice.org.uk/guidance/ng206 [Accessed 2024].

The ME Society (2023), 'Long Covid and ME/CFS Are they the same condition?' meassociation.org.uk/wp-content/uploads/LONG-COVID-AND-MECFS-ARE-THEY-THE-SAME-CONDITION-MAY-2023.pdf [Accessed 2024].

NICE. Clinical Knowledge Summaries (2024), 'Anaemia – iron deficiency'. cks.nice.org.uk/topics/anaemia-iron-deficiency [Accessed 2024].

Chapter 6

NICE. Clinical Knowledge Summaries (2024), 'Menorrhagia (heavy menstrual bleeding)'. cks.nice.org.uk/topics/menorrhagia-heavy-menstrual-bleeding [Accessed 2024].

British Menopause Society. 'Management of unscheduled bleeding on hormone replacement therapy (HRT)'. thebms.org.uk/wp-content/uploads/2024/12/01-BMS-GUIDELINE-Management-of-unscheduled-bleeding-HRT-NOVEMBER2024-A.pdf [Accessed 2025]

Lenart-Lipińska, M., Matyjaszek-Matuszek, B., Woźniakowska, E., Solski, J., Tarach, J.S., Paszkowski, T. (2014), 'Polycystic ovary syndrome: clinical implication in perimenopause'. *Przeglad Menopauzalny/Menopause Review*, 13(6):348–351.

Jefferies, K., Bland, L., Oladimeji, B., et al. (2024), 'Uterine fibroids and Black people of African descent globally: a scoping review protocol'. *BMJ Open* 14:e085622. doi.org/10.1136/bmjopen-2024-085622.

Ulin, M., Ali, M., Chaudhry, Z.T., Al-Hendy, A., Yang, Q. (2020), 'Uterine fibroids in menopause and perimenopause'. *Menopause*, 27(2):238–242.

NICE Guideline [NG88] (2018 – updated 2021), 'Heavy menstrual bleeding: assessment and management'. nice.org.uk/guidance/ng88 [Accessed 2025].

NICE Clinical Knowledge Summaries (2023), 'Fibroids'. cks.nice.org.uk/topics/fibroids [Accessed 2025].

Chapter 7

Amit, G. (2014), 'Breast Pain'. *BMJ Clinical Evidence* ncbi.nlm.nih.gov/pmc/articles/PMC4200534 [Accessed 2024].

Scurr, J., Hedger, W., Morris, P., Brown, N. (2014), 'The prevalence, severity and impact of breast pain in the general population'. *The Breast Journal*, 20(5):508–513.

Brown, N., White, J., Brasher, A., et al. (2014), 'The experience of breast pain (mastalgia) in female runners of the 2012 London Marathon and its effect on exercise behaviour'. *British Journal of Sports Medicine,* 48:320–325.

White, J., Scurr, J. (2012), 'Evaluation of professional bra fitting criteria for bra selection and fitting in the UK'. *Ergonomics,* 55(6):704–711.

Hubbard, T.J.E., Sharma, A., Ferguson, D.J. (2020), 'Breast pain: assessment, management and referral criteria'. *British Journal of General Practice,* 70(697):419–420.

Hafiz, S.P., Barnes, N.L.P., Kirwan, C. (2018), 'Clinical management of idiopathic mastalgia: a systematic review'. *Journal of Primary Health Care,* 10, 312–323.

Scurr, J.C., White, J.L., Hedger, W. (2011), 'Supported and unsupported breast displacement in three dimensions across treadmill activity levels'. *Journal of Sports Sciences,* Jan:29(1):55–61. doi.org/10.1080/02640414.2010.521944.

NICE guideline [CG164] (2013), 'Familial breast cancer: classification, care and managing breast cancer and related risks in people with a family history of breast cancer'. nice.org.uk/guidance/cg164/chapter/recommendations [Accessed 2024].

Bruning, P.F., Bonfrèr, J.M., van Noord, P.A., Hart, A.A., de Jong-Bakker, M., Nooijen, W.J. (1992), 'Insulin resistance and breast-cancer risk'. *International Journal of Cancer,* Oct 21;52(4):511–6. doi.org/10.1002/ijc.2910520402.

Rose, D.P., Gracheck, P.J., Vona-Davis, L. (2015), 'The interactions of Obesity, Inflammation and Insulin Resistance in Breast Cancer'. *Cancers,* 7(4):2146–2168. doi.org/10.3390/cancers/7040883.

Chapter 8

Elia, G., Bergman, A. (1993), 'Estrogen effects on the urethra: beneficial effects in women with genuine stress incontinence'. *Obstetrical Gynecological Survey,* 48(7):509–517.

Robinson, D. (2024), 'Oestrogens and lower urinary tract dysfunction chronicling a lifetime of research'. *Continence,* 12, 101720.

Carlson, K., Nguyen, H. (2024), 'Genitourinary Syndrome of Menopause'. *StatPearls,* ncbi.nlm.nih.gov/books/NBK559297 [Accessed 2025].

British Society for Sexual Medicine. 'Position Statement for Management of Genitourinary Syndrome of the Menopause (GSM)'. bssm.org.uk/wp-content/uploads/2023/02/GSM-BSSM.pdf [Accessed 2025].

NICE Guidance. (2015 – updated 2021), 'Urinary incontinence in women' nice.org.uk/guidance/qs77 [Accessed 2025].

Chapter 9

Peters, B.A., Santoro, N., Kaplan, R.C., & Qi, Q. (2022), 'Spotlight on the Gut Microbiome in Menopause: Current Insights'. *International Journal of Women's Health,* 14, 1059–1072. doi.org/10.2147/IJWH.S340491.

Boytar, A.N., Skinner, T.L., Wallen, R.E., Jenkins, D.G., Dekker Nitert, M. (2023), 'The Effect of Exercise Prescription on the Human Gut Microbiota and Comparison between Clinical and Apparently Healthy Populations: A Systematic Review'. *Nutrients,* 22;15(6):1534.

NICE Clinical guideline [CG61]. (2008 – updated 2017), 'Irritable bowel syndrome in adults: diagnosis and management'. nice.org.uk/guidance/cg61 [Accessed 2025].

Stachenfeld, N.S. (2014), 'Hormonal changes during menopause and the impact on fluid regulation'. *Reproductive Sciences,* 21(5):555–561.

Jung, H.K., Choung, R.S., Talley, N.J. (2010), 'Gastroesophageal reflux disease and sleep disroders: evidence for a causal link and therapeutic implications'. *Journal of Neurogastroenterology and Motility,* 16(1):22–29.

Infantino, M. (2008), 'The prevalence and pattern of gastroesophageal reflux symptoms in perimenopausal and menopausal women'. *Journal of the American Academy of Nurse Practitioners,* 20:266–272.

NICE guideline [NG151]. (2020 – updated 2021), 'Colorectal cancer'. nice.org.uk/guidance/ng151 [Accessed 2025].

NICE. Clinical Knowledge Summaries, 'Ovarian Cancer'. cks.nice.org.uk/topics/ovarian-cancer [Accessed 2025].

Chapter 10

Ram Hong, A., Wan Kim, S. (2018), 'Effects of Resistance Exercise on Bone Health', *Endocrinology and Metabolism,* 33(4):435–444.

Holden, M.A., Hattle, M., Runhaar, J., et al. (2023), 'Moderators of the effect of therapeutic exercise for knee and hip osteoarthritis: a systematic review and individual participant data meta-analysis' *The Lancet Rheumatology,* 5(7):e386-e400.

Lo, G.H., Driban, J.B., Kriska, A.M., McAlindon, T.E., Souza, R.B., Petersen, N.J., Storki, K.L., Eaton, C.B., Hochberg, M.C., Jackson, R.D., Kent, K.C., Nevitt, M.C., Suarez-Almazor, M.E. (2017), 'Is There an Association Between a History of Running and Symptomatic Knee Osteoarthritis? A Cross-Sectional Study From the Osteoarthritis Initiative'. *Arthritis Care Res (Hoboken),* Feb;69(2):183–191. doi.org/10.1002/acr.22939.

Lo, G.H., Musa, S.M., Driban, J.B., Kriska, A.M., McAlindon, T.E., Souza, R.B., Petersen, N.J., Storti, K.L., Eaton, C.B., Hochberg, M.C., Jackson, R.D., Kwoh, C.K., Nevitt, M.C., Suarez-Almazor, M.E. (2018), 'Running does not increase symptoms or structural progression in people with knee osteoarthritis: data from the osteoarthritis initiative'. *Clinical Rheumatology,* 37(9):2497–2504. doi.org/10.1007/s10067-018-4121-3.

Alentorn-Geli, E., Samuelson, K., Musahl, V., Green, C.L., Bhandari, M., Karlsson, J. (2017) 'The Association of Recreational and Competitive Running with Hip and Knee Osteoarthritis: A systematic Review and Meta-analysis'. *Journal of Orthopaedic & Sports Physical Therapy,* 47(6):373–390. doi.org/10.2519/jospt.2017.7137.

Brooke-Wavell, K., Skelton, D.A., Barker, K.L. et al, (2022), 'Strong, steady and straight: UK consensus statement on physical activity and exercise for osteoporosis'. *British Journal of Sports Medicine,* 56:837–846.

Fang, Y., Liu, F., Zhang, X., Chen, L., Liu, Y., Yang, L., Zheng, X., Liu, J., Li, K., Li, Z. (2024), 'Mapping global prevalence of menopausal symptoms among middle-aged women: a systematic review and meta-analysis'. *BMC Public Health,* 24(1):1767.

Haines, C.J., Xing, S.M., Park, K.H., Holinka, C.F. Ausmanas, M.K. (2005), 'Prevalence of menopausal symptoms in different ethnic groups of Asian women and responsiveness to therapy with three doses of conjugated estrogens/medoxyprogesterone acetate: the Pan-Asia Menopause (PAM) study'. *Maturitas,* 52(3-4):261–276. doi.org/10.1016/j.maturitas.2005.03.012.

Khalid, A.B., Krum, S.A. (2016), 'Estrogen receptors alpha and beta in bone'. *Bone,* 87:130-5.

Dennison, E.M. (2022), 'Osteoarthritis: The importance of hormonal status in midlife women'. *Maturitas,* 165: 8–11.

Chidi-Ogbolu, N., Baar, K. (2019), 'Effect of Estrogen on Musculoskeletal Performance and Injury Risk'. *Frontiers in Physiology,* 15;9:1834.

NICE guideline [NG226], (2022), 'Osteoarthritis in over 16s: diagnosis and management'. nice.org.uk/guidance/ng226 [Accessed 2024].

Chapter 11

Lu, C., Liu, P., Zhou, Y., Meng, F., Qiao, T., Yang, X., Li, X., Xue, Q., Xu, H., Liu, Y., Zhang, Y. (2020), 'Musculoskeletal Pain during the Menopausal Transition: A Systematic Review and Meta-Analysis'. *Neural Plasticity,* 25:8842110.

Bettariga, F., Taaffe, D., Galvão, D.A., Lopez, P., Bishop, C., Markarian, A.M., Natalucci, V., Kim, J.S., Newton, R.U. (2024), 'Exercise training mode effects on myokine expression in healthy adults: A systematic review with meta-analysis'. *Journal of Sport and Health Science,* 16:6:764–779.

Peeters, G., van Schoor, N.M., Cooper, R., Tooth, L., Kenny, R.A. (2018), 'Should prevention of falls start earlier? Co-ordinated analyses of harmonised data on falls in middle-aged adults across four population-based cohort studies'. *Plos One,* doi.org/10.1371/journal.pone.0201989 [Accessed 2024].

Walston, J.D. (2012), 'Sarcopenia in older adults'. *Current Opinion in Rheumatology,* 24(6):623–627.

Macfarlane, G.J., Beasey, M., Jones E.A., et al. (2012), 'The prevalence and management of low back pain across adulthood: results from a population-based cross-sectional study (the MUSICIAN study)'. *Pain,* 153(1): 27–32.

Adera, T., Deyo, R.A., Donatelle, R.J. (1994), 'Premature menopause and low back pain. A population-based study'. *Annals of Epidemiology,* 4(5):416–422.

Yip, Y., Ho, S.C., Chan, S. (2002), 'Socio-psychological stressors as risk factors for low back pain in Chinese middle-aged women'. *Journal of Advanced Nursing,* 36(3):409–416.

Nikolov, V., Petkova, M. (2010), 'Pain sensitivity among women with low oestrogen levels'. *Procedia,* 5:289–293.

Maffulli, N., Cuozzo, F., Migliorini, F., et al. (2023), 'The tendon unit: biochemical, biomechanical, hormonal influences'. *Journal of Orthopaedic Surgery and Research,* 18:311. doi.org/10.1186/s13018-023-03796-4.

NICE guideline [NG59]. (2016), 'Low back pain and sciatica in over 16s: assessment and management'. nice.org.uk/guidance/ng59 [Accessed 2024].

The Royal Orthopaedic Hospital, 'Gluteal tendinopathy'. roh.nhs.uk/services-information/therapy/gluteal-tendinopathy [Accessed 2024].

Cowan, R.M., Ganderton, C.L., Cook, J., Semciw, A.I., Long, D.M., Pizzari, T. (2022), 'Does Menopausal Hormone Therapy, Exercise or Both Improve Pain and Function in Post-menopausal Women With Greater Trochanteric Pain Syndrome? A 2x2 Factorial Randomized, Clinical Trial'. *The American Journal of Sports Medicine,* 50(2):515–525.

Sipilä, S., Törmäkangas, T., Sillanpää, E., Aukee, P., Kujala, U.M., Kovanen, V., Laakkonen, E.K. (2020), 'Muscle and bone mass in middle-aged women: role of menopausal status and physical activity'. *Journal of Cachexia Sarcopenia Muscle,* 11(3):698–709. doi.org/10.1002/jcsm.12547.

Chapter 12

Greendale, G.A., Sternfeld, B., Huang, M., Han, W., Karvonen-Gutierrez, C., Ruppert, K., Cauley, J.A., Finkelstein, J.S., Jiang, S., Karlamangla, A.S. (2019), 'Changes in body composition and weight during the menopause transition'. *JCI Insight,* 4(5):e124865. doi.org/10.1172/jci.insight.124865.

Hurtado, M.D., Saadedine, M., Kapoor, E., Shufelt, C.L., Faubion, S. (2024), 'Weight Gain in Midlife Women'. *Current Obesity Reports,* 13(2):352–363. doi.org/10.1007/s13679-024-00555-2.

Ambikairajah, A., Walsh, E., Tabatabaei-Jafari, H., Cherbuin, N. (2019), 'Fat mass changes during menopause: a metaanalysis'. *American Journal of Obstetrics Gynecology,* 221(5):393-409. doi.org/10.1016/j.ajog.2019.04.023.

Patel, S.R., Malhotra, A., White, D.P., Gottlieb, D.J., Hu, F.B. (2006), 'Association between reduced sleep and weight gain in women'. *American Journal of Epidemiology,* 164(10):947-954. doi.org/10.1093/aje/kwj280.

Cappuccio, F.P., D'Elia, L., Strazzullo, P., Miller, M.A. (2010), 'Sleep duration and all-cause mortality: a systematic review and meta-analysis of prospective studies'. *Sleep,* 33(5):585-92. doi.org/10.1093/sleep/33.5.585.

Zaidi, M., Lizneva, D., Kim, S.M., Sun, L., Iqbal, J., New, M.I., Rosen, C.J., Yuen, T. (2018), 'FSH, Bone Mass, Body Fat, and Biological Aging', *Endocrinology,* 159(10):3503–3514. doi.org/10.1210/en.2018-00601.

Kadowaki, T., Yamauchi, T., Kubota, N., Hara, K., Ueki, K., Tobe, K. (2006), 'Adiponectin and adiponectin receptors in insulin resistance, diabetes, and the metabolic syndrome'. *Journal of Clinical Investigation,* 116(7):1784–1792. doi.org/10.1172/JCI29126

Chandran, M., Phillips, S.A., Ciaraldi, T., Henry, R.R. (2003), 'Adiponectin: More Than Just Another Fat Cell Hormone?' *Diabetes Care* 26 (8):2442–2450. doi.org/10.2337/diacare.26.8.2442.

Khoramipour, K., Chamari, K., Hekmatikar, A.A., Ziyaiyan, A., Taherkhani, S., Elguindy, N.M., Bragazzi, N.L. (2021), 'Adiponectin: Structure, Physiological Functions, Role in Diseases and Effects of Nutrition'. *Nutrients,* 13(4):1180. doi.org/10.3390/nu13041180.

Mankowska, A., Nowak, L., Sypniewska, G. (2009), 'Adiponectin and Metabolic Syndrome in Women at Menopause'. *eJIFCC,* 19(4):173–184.

Wu, Y., Zheng, C., Chen, D., Xie, M. (2015), 'Investigation of the change of adiponectin level with menopause status in middle aged women and its relationship with androgen'. *Zhonghua Fu Chan Ke Za Zhi.* 50(5):356–360.

British Menopause Society. (2023), 'Menopause: Nutrition and Weight Gain'. thebms.org.uk/wp-content/uploads/2023/06/19-BMS-TfC-Menopause-Nutrition-and-Weight-Gain-JUNE2023-A.pdf [Accessed 2025].

Ambikairajah, A., Walsh, E., Tabatabaei-Jafari, H., Cherbuin, N. (2019), 'Fat mass changes during menopause: a metaanalysis'. *Am J Obstet Gynecol,* 221(5):393–409.e50. doi.org/10.1016/j.ajog.2019.04.023.

Chapter 13

Falcone, D., Richters, R.J., Uzunbajakava, N.E., Van Erp, P.E., Van de Kerkhof, P.C. (2017), 'Sensitive skin and the influence of female hormone fluctuation: results from a cross-sectional digital survey in the Dutch population'. *European Journal of Dermatology,* 27(1):42–48.

Rzepecki, A., Murase, J.E., Juran, R., Fabi, S.G., McLellan, B.N. (2019), 'Estrogen-deficient skin: The role of topical therapy'. *International Journal of Women's Dermatology.* Mar 15;5(2):85–90.

NICE guidelines [NG14]. (2014 – updated 2022), 'Melanoma: assessment and management'. nice.org.uk/guidance/ng14 [Accessed 2024].

Findlay, Q., Reid, K. (2018), 'Dry eye disease: when to treat and when to refer'. *Australian Prescriber,* 41(5):160–163. doi.org/10.18773/austprescr.2018.048.

Chapter 14

Mosconi, L., Berti, V., Dyke, J., et al. (2021), 'Menopause impacts human brain structure, connectivity, energy metabolism, and amylod-beta deposition'. *Scientific Reports,* 11, 10867.

Mosconi, L., Nerattini, M., Matthews, D.C., et al. (2024), 'In vivo brain estrogen receptor density by neuroendocrine aging and relationships with cognition and symptomatology'. *Scientific Reports* 14, 12680.

Bromberger, J.T., Kravitz, H.M., Yuefang, C., Randolph, J.F., jr. Avis, N.E., Gold, E B., Matthews, K.A. (2013), 'Does risk for anxiety increase during the menopausal transition? Study of Women's Health Across the Nation'. *Menopause* 20(5): 488–495. doi.org/10.1097/gme.0b013e3182730599.

Shitomi-Jones, L.M., Dolman, C., Jones, I., et al. (2024), 'Exploration of first onsets of mania, schizophrenia spectrum disorders and major depressive disorder in perimenopause'. *Nature Mental Health.* doi.org/10.1038/s44220-024-00292-4.

Badaway, Y., Spector, A., Li, Z., Desai, R. (2024), 'The risk of depression in the menopausal stages: A systematic review and meta-analysis'. *Journal of Affective Disorders* 357: 126–133.

Woldeamanuel, Y.W., Oliveira, A.B.D. (2022), 'What is the efficacy of aerobic exercise versus strength training in the treatment of migraine? A systematic review and network meta-analysis of clinical trials'. *Journal of Headache and Pain* 23, 134. doi.org/10.1186/s10194-022-01503-y.

La Touche, R., Fierro-Marrero, J., Sánchez-Ruíz, I., et al. (2023), 'Prescription of therapeutic exercise in migraine, an evidence-based clinical practice guideline'. *Journal of Headache and Pain* 24, 68. doi.org/10.1186/s10194-023-01571-8.

Karimi, L., Wijeratne, T., Crewther, S.G., Evans, A., Ebaid, D, Khalil, H. (2020), 'The Migraine-Anxiety Comorbidity Among Migraineurs: A Systematic Review'. *Frontiers in Neurology* 11. doi.org/10.3389/fneur.2020.613372

Chapter 15

British Menopause Society – HRT Guide. (2022), thebms.org.uk/wp-content/uploads/2022/12/04-BMS-TfC-HRT-Guide-NOV2022-A.pdf [Accessed 2025].

British Menopause Society – Consensus Statement. (2020), 'BMS and WHC's 2020 recommendations on hormone replacement therapy in menopausal women'. thebms.org.uk/wp-content/uploads/2023/10/02-BMS-ConsensusStatement-BMS-WHC-2020-Recommendations-on-HRT-in-menopausal-women-SEPT2023-A.pdf [Accessed 2025].

Panay, N., Ang, S.B., Cheshire, R., Goldstein, S.R., Maki, P., Nappi, R.E., and on behalf of the International Menopause Society Board. (2024), 'Menopause and MHT in 2024: addressing the key controversies – an International Menopause Society White Paper'. *Climacteric*. doi.org/10.1080/13697137.2024.2394950.

NHS Business Services Authority. (2024), 'Hormone Replacement Therapy – England, April 2015 to June 2024'. cms.nhsbsa.nhs.uk/statistical-collections/hormone-replacement-therapy-england/hormone-replacement-therapy-england-april-2015-june-2024 [Accessed 2024].

NICE guideline [NG23]. (2024), 'Menopause: identification and management'. nice.org.uk/guidance/NG23 [Accessed 2024].

NICE. Clinical Knowledge Summaries. (2024), 'Hormone Replacement Therapy (HRT)'. cks.nice.org.uk/topics/menopause/prescribing-information/hormone-replacement-therapy-hrt [Accessed 2025].

Women's Health Concern. (2019), 'Breast cancer risk factors'. womens-health-concern.org/wp-content/uploads/2022/12/01-WHC-FACTSHEET-BreastCancer-NOV2022-C.pdf [Accessed 2024].

Women's Health Concern (2020), 'HRT: The history'. womens-health-concern.org/wp-content/uploads/2022/11/10-WHC-FACTSHEET-HRT-The-history-NOV22-A.pdf [Accessed 2024].

Cho, M.K. (2018), 'Use of Combined Oral Contraceptives in Perimenopausal Women'. *Chonnam Medical Journal,* 54(3):153–158.

The Faculty of Sexual and Reproductive Healthcare. (2017 – updated 2023), 'FSRH Guideline: Contraception for Women Aged Over 40 Years'. fsrh.org/Common/Uploaded%20files/documents/fsrh-guideline-contraception-for-women-aged-over-40-years-august-2017-amended-july-2023-.pdf [Accessed 2025].

British Menopause Society. 'Prescribable alternatives to HRT'. thebms.org.uk/wp-content/uploads/2018/03/Prescribable-alternatives-to-HRT-01EE.pdf [Accessed 2025].

Nguyen, M. (2013), 'The use of pregabalin in the treatment of hot flashes'. *Canadian Pharmacists Journal*, 146(4):193–196.

Kam-Hansen, S., Jakubowski, M., Kelley, J.M., Kirsch, I., Hoaglin, D.C., Kaptchuk, T.J., Burstein, R. (2014), 'Altered placebo and drug labeling changes the outcome of episodic migraine attacks'. Sci Transl Med. 2014 6(218):218ra5. doi.org/10.1126/scitranslmed.3006175.

British Menopause Society. Consensus statement. (2024), 'Non-hormonal-based treatments for menopausal symptoms'. thebms.org.uk/wp-content/uploads/2024/09/04-BMS-ConsensusStatement-Non-hormonal-based-treatments-SEPT2024-A.pdf [Accessed 2025].

L'Espérance, S., Frenette, S., Dionne, A., Dionne, J.Y. Comité de l'évolution des pratiques en oncologie (CEPO). (2013), 'Pharmacological and non-hormonal treatment of hot flashes in breast cancer survivors: CEPO review and recommendations'. *Supportive Care in Cancer*. 21(5):1461–1474. doi.org/10.1007/s00520-013-1732-8.

Rada, G., Capurro, D., Pantoja, T., Corbalán, J., Moreno, G., Letelier, L.M., Vera, C. (2010), 'Non-hormonal interventions for hot flushes in women with a history of breast cancer'. *Cochrane Database of Systematic Reviews* Issue 9. Art. No.: CD004923. doi.org/10.1002/14651858.CD004923.pub2.

Villaseca, P. (2012), 'Non-estrogen conventional and phytochemical treatments for vasomotor symptoms: what needs to be known for practice'. *Climacteric*. 2012 15(2):115–124. doi.org/10.3109/13697137.2011.624214.

National Institutes of Health. Office of Dietary Supplements. 'Black Cohosh. Fact Sheet for Health Professionals'. ods.od.nih.gov/factsheets/BlackCohosh-HealthProfessional [Accessed 2025].

Women's Health Concern. (2024), 'Complementary & alternative therapies. Non hormonal treatments for menopause symptoms'. womens-health-concern.org/wp-content/uploads/2024/11/03-WHC-FACTSHEET-Complementary-And-Alternative-Therapies-NOV2024-B.pdf [Accessed 2024].

Lund, K.S., Siersma, V., Brodersen, J., et al. (2018), 'Efficacy of a standardised acupuncture approach for women with bothersome menopausal symptoms: a pragmatic randomised study in primary care (the ACOM study)'. BMJ Open 9:e023637. doi.org/10.1136/bmjopen-2018-023637.

Moffet, H.H. (2009), 'Sham acupuncture may be as efficacious as true acupuncture: a systematic review of clinical trials'. *The Journal of Alternative and Complementary Medicine*, 15(3):213–6. doi.org/10.1089/acm.2008.0356.

Chapter 16

Gröber, U., Werner, T., Vormann, J., Kisters, K. (2017), 'Myth or Reality – Transdermal Magnesium?' *Nutrients,* 9(8):813.

Calder, P. (2017), 'New evidence that omega-3 fatty acids have a role in primary prevention of coronary heart disease'. *Journal of Public Health and Emergency,* 1(2). doi.org/10.21037/jphe.2017.03.03.

NHS. 'Vitamins and minerals'. nhs.uk/conditions/vitamins-and-minerals [Accessed 2025].

Welton, S., Minty, R., O'Driscoll, T., Willms, H., Poirier, D., Madden, S., Kelly, L. (2020), 'Intermittent fasting and weight loss: Systematic review'. *Canadian Family Physician,* 66(2):117–125.

Cone-Pipo, J., Mora-Fernandez, A., Martinez-Bebia, M., Gimenez-Blasi, N., Lopez-Moro, A., Latorre, J.A., Almendros-Ruiz, A., Requena, B., Mariscal-Arcas, M. (2024), 'Intermittent Fasting: Does It Affect Sports Performance? A Systematic Review'. *Nutrients,* 4;16(1):168. doi.org/10.3390/nu16010168.

Maruthur, N.M., Pilla, S.J., White, K., Wu, B., Maw, M.T.T., Duan, D., Turkson-Ocran, R.A., Zhao, D., Charleston, J., Peterson, C.M., Dougherty, R.J., Schrack, J.A., Appel, L.J., Guallar, E., Clark, J.M. (2024), 'Effect of Isocaloric, Time-Restricted Eating on Body Weight in Adults With Obesity: A Randomized Controlled Trial'. *Annals of Internal Medicine,* 177(5):549–558. doi.org/10.7326/M23-3132.

Cronin, O., Lanham-New, S.A., Corfe, B.M., et al. (2022), 'Role of the Microbiome in Regulating Bone Metabolism and Susceptibility to Osteoporosis'. *Calcified Tissue International,* 110(3): 273–284.

de Miranda, R.B. Weimer, P. Rossi, R.C. (2021), 'Effects of hydrolysed collagen supplementation on skin aging: a systematic review and meta-analysis'. *International Journal of Dermatology,* 60(12):1449–1461.

Smith-Ryan, A.E., Cabre, H.E., Eckerson, J.M., Candow, D.G. (2021), 'Creatine Supplementation in Women's Health: A Lifespan Perspective'. *Nutrients,* 13(3): 877.

Chapters 17–19

Boutcher, Y.N., Boutcher, S.H., Yoo, H.Y., Meerkin, J.D. (2019), 'The Effect of Sprint Interval Training on Body Composition of Post-menopausal Women'. *Medicine and Science in Sports and Exercise,* 51(7):1413–1419.

Maillard, F., Rousset, S., Pereira, B., Traore, A., de Pradel Del Amaze, P., Boirie, Y., Duclos, M., Boisseau, N. (2016), 'High-intensity interval training reduces abdominal fat mass in post-menopausal women with type 2 diabetes'. *Diabetes and Metabolism Journal,* 42(6):433–441.

Jones, A.M., Doust, J.H. (1996), 'A 1% treadmill grade most accurately reflects the energetic cost of outdoor running'. *Journal of Sports Science,* 14(4):321–7. doi.org/10.1080/02640419608727717.

Ramesh, S., James, M.T., Holroyd-Leduc, J.M., Wilton, S.B., Sola, D.Y., Ahmed, S.B. (2022), 'Heart rate variability as a function of menopausal status, menstrual cycle phase and estradiol level'. *Physiological Reports,* 10(10):e15298. doi.org/10.14814/phy2.15298.

Gilani, M.A., Ghumatkar, M., Kumar, A. (2020), 'Comparison of VO2 Max between Natural and Surgical Post-menopausal Women'. 10(6).

Gurjão, A.L., Gonçalves, R., de Moura, R.F., Gobbi, S. (2009), 'Acute effect of static stretching on rate of force development and maximal voluntary contraction in older women'. *The Journal of Strength and Conditioning Research,* 23(7):2149–2154. doi.org/10.1519/JSC.0b013e3181b8682d.

Capel-Alcaraz, A.M., García-López, H., Castro-Sánchez, A.M., Fernández-Sánchez, M., Lara-Palomo, I.C. (2023), 'The Efficacy of Strength Exercises for Reducing the Symptoms of Menopause: A Systematic Review'. *Journal of Clinical Medicine,* 12(2):548. doi.org/10.3390/jcm12020548.

Svensen, E., Koscien, C.P., Alamdari, N., Wall, B.T., Stephens, F.B. (2025), 'A Novel Low-Impact Resistance Exercise Program Increases Strength and Balance in Females Irrespective of Menopause Status'. *Medicine & Science in Sports & Exercise* 57(3):501–513. doi.org/10.1249/MSS.0000000000003586.

Index

Note: Entries for menopause, excluding post-menopause, also relate to perimenopause.

aches and pains *see* joint pain; muscle health; periods
Achilles tendinopathy 117
acupuncture 176
adenomyosis 50, 56
adiponectin 127
adrenal fatigue 46
adrenal glands 5
alcohol consumption 33, 66, 95, 154, 165
Alzheimer's disease 13, 152
anaemia 42–3, 55, 190
anovulatory cycles 5, 50
antidepressants 151, 154, 171–2, 174
anxiety 17, 45, 55, 145, 148–9, 154, 155, 160, 171, 172
   see also mental health
appetite 123, 179
arthritis 96, 98
autoimmune conditions 44–5

back pain 113–14
balance and coordination 14, 106, 209–10, 274
basal metabolic rate (BMR) 123
bipolar disorder 144
black cohosh 174
bladder issues 18, 33
blood loss 52–5, 164
body composition changes 120–2
   action steps 131
   causes 122–4
   impact of HRT 130
   sedentary time 128–30
   subcutaneous fat 125, 126
   visceral fat 125, 126–7, 129, 130
   waist-to-hip and waist-to-height ratios 128
bone health 13, 56, 91–7, 181
bowel conditions 95
brain fog/forgetfulness 18, 151
brain function, human 4–5, 20, 29, 147, 152, 181
bras, sports 61, 63–4, 134
breasts
   cancer 65–7, 160, 165, 172, 174
   looking after your 66
   menopause and structural changes 62–3
   pain and tenderness 17, 58–61, 167
   sports bras 61, 63–4
   treatments for 61–2
   when to see your doctor 62

caffeine 32–3, 154, 189
calorie intake 180, 184, 197
cancer 13, 51, 65–6, 105, 140, 160, 164, 165, 171, 174
carpal tunnel syndrome 120
chafing 133–4

chemical menopause 55
chest pain 26–7
Chinese medicine 175
chronic systemic inflammation 105–6, 108
cognitive behavioural therapy (CBT) 25, 35, 154, 171
collagen 103, 104, 110, 132, 137, 194–5, 196
contraception 10–11, 53–4, 153, 169
   combined oral contraceptives 11, 54, 153, 169–70
cortisol 46, 123–4, 147–8
cramp 112, 168
creatine 194, 195

deep vein thrombosis (DVT) 163, 164
depression 148, 150, 154, 155, 171
diabetes 13, 51, 105, 106, 124, 127
diagnosis of menopause and perimenopause 9–10, 12
diet *see* nutrition
differing experiences 6, 8, 17–18
dizziness/light-headedness 42
dry eye disease 137
dysfunctional uterine bleeding (DUB) 50

early menopause 6, 10, 95, 158
electrolyte imbalance 112
endometrial ablation 55
endometrial hyperplasia 51
endometriosis 50, 51–2, 56
endurance events 53
energy levels 37, 180–1, 189
   adrenal fatigue 46
   impact of menopause symptoms 37–8
   lifestyle factors 38
      movement 39
      nutrition 39, 180–2, 185
      relaxation 40–1
      sleep 40
      social health and connection 41–2
   managing 47–8
   medical conditions 42–5, 46
   mental health issues 45
   when to see your doctor 46–7
ethnicity and menopause 6, 18, 51, 90, 121
evening primrose oil 175
eye health 138, 140

facial hair 133, 166
falls, danger of 14, 106
fat, body 63, 65, 106, 107, 120–31
fatigue *see* energy levels
fats, dietary 186, 188
fertility loss 40, 49, 146
fibroids 50–1, 56
fibromyalgia 110–11
follicle-stimulating hormone (FSH) 4, 5, 10, 21, 29, 123, 127
foot health 137

324   The Runner's Guide to Menopause

gluteal tendinopathy 117–18
gonadotropin-releasing hormone (GnRH) 4–5
gut microbiome 193

heart disease 13, 14, 105, 164
heart rate 42, 205, 218–19
hormone tests 10, 11
hot flushes/night sweats 17, 18, 19, 160–1
   cause of 20–1
   effect on running 21–2
   medical treatments 24, 171–3
   self-help 23
   supplements and herbal remedies 25, 175
   when to see your doctor 26–7
HRT (hormone replacement therapy) 11, 21, 24, 35, 45, 51, 53–4, 62, 97, 104, 109, 115, 130, 137, 151, 153, 154, 158, 172–3
   body identical and bioidentical hormones 162–3
   impact on running 167–8
   patches, gels and exercise 168–9
   risks of HRT 164–5
   side-effects 167–8
   testosterone 166–7
   types of 162–4, 166–7, 168–9
   using contraception 169–70
   vaginal oestrogen 170
   what symptoms will HRT improve? 160
   what symptoms with HRT not improve? 160–1
   when it doesn't work 165–6
   when to consider 158
   when to start taking 161–2
   when to stop taking? 162
   who can't take HRT? 159
   who doesn't need HRT? 159
hunger 179–80
hyperthyroidism (overactive thyroid) 44–5
hypothalamic-pituitary-ovarian axis 5
hypothalamus 4–5, 20–1
hypothyroidism (underactive thyroid) 44, 45
hysterectomy 7, 55

identity, loss of 145
incontinence 114
inflammation 65, 101, 103, 105–6, 108, 110, 115, 126, 129
insulin resistance 106, 127
intertrigo 135
intrauterine system (IUS)/coils 53–4

joint pain 18, 90, 98–104
jumping drills 92

libido 18, 51, 166
ligaments 102, 110
luteinising hormone (LH) 4, 5, 21

medical menopause 7
medications 24, 35–6, 44, 45, 51, 53–4, 56, 61, 94, 96, 97, 153, 154–5, 163, 172–3
   see also HRT (hormone replacement therapy)
mefenamic acid 53
melatonin 29

menorrhagia see periods
menstrual cycle 4
mental health 13, 18, 45, 49
   anxiety 17, 45, 55, 145, 148, 154, 155, 160–1
   brain fog 151
   depression 148, 150, 154, 155
   how running can help 155–6
   lifestyle steps to improve 153–4
   medical treatment 154–5
   menopause and brain changes 147
   menopause life changes 146
   menopause symptoms 143–4
   running and menopause symptoms 144–5
   when to see your doctor 150
   see also stress
metabolism 107
micronutrients see omega-3 fatty acids; vitamins and minerals
migraines 152–3
mindset, positive 302
   believe in yourself 303
   consistency is key 304
   getting started 306–9
   keep learning 304
   making changes 305
   unnecessary pressure 303
muscle health
   and balance 106
   common problems 18, 90, 109–14
   mass and sarcopenia 13, 107–9, 130, 270
   and metabolism 107
   role of myokines 105–6
   see also strength training
musculoskeletal syndrome of menopause 18, 90–104
   bone health 91–7
   joint pain 98–104
   muscle health 105–14
   osteoporosis 94–7
   tendon health 115–19
   when to see your doctor 95–6, 100, 114
myalgia 109
   see also muscle health
myokines 105–6, 129

night sweats see hot flushes/night sweats
non-steroidal anti-inflammatories (NSAIDs) 53, 56, 61, 110
norethisterone 54, 55
nutrition 39, 93, 108–9, 206
   anti-inflammatory foods 104
   avoiding hunger 179–80, 197
   calorie intake 180, 184, 197
   carbohydrates 184, 186–7
   choosing quality foods 186, 197
   collagen and creatine 194–5
   common menopause related complaints 178–9
   dietary iron 43, 189
   eating after a run 185
   eating before a run 182–3
   eating during a run 184
   energy levels 180–2

fats 186, 188
fibre 193–4
gut microbiome 193
intermittent fasting (IF) 184
macronutrients 186–7
mental health 153, 154
phytoestrogens and isoflavones 173–4
protein 109, 186–7
timing your eating 182–4
tracking apps 192
treatment for breast pain 61
see also body composition changes; vitamins and minerals

obesity 21, 115, 165
oestrogen levels 4–5, 8, 14, 21, 29, 51, 62, 65, 81, 85, 90, 99, 102, 103, 111, 115, 123, 127, 132, 133, 136, 139, 147, 160, 162, 163, 170, 179
'old women' stereotype, menopause and 8
omega-3 fatty acids 104, 191
osteoarthritis 98–9
osteoclasts 92
osteoporosis 13, 93, 94–7, 98, 128
ovarian follicle production 4, 6
ovulation 4, 5

painkillers 53, 56, 61, 94, 109, 110, 111, 119
palpitations 26–7, 42, 154, 161
periods 4–5, 42–3, 96, 189
  breast pain 59–60
  consequences of heavy 55
  delaying with norethisterone 55
  heavy and painful during perimenopause 49–52
  identifying menopause 55
  impacting running 57
  lack of 56
  managing heavy periods 52–5
  painful 56
  when to see your doctor 57
Pilates 113, 273
piriformis syndrome 114
pituitary gland 4–5, 10, 95
placebo effect 173, 174–5
plantar fasciitis 103
plyometrics 204, 274
polycystic ovary syndrome (PCOS) 6, 50, 51
post-menopause 7, 50, 60, 164
posture 97, 106
pregnancy 4, 96
premature menopause 6–7, 10, 40, 95, 158
probiotics 193
progesterone levels 4–5, 29, 51, 53–4, 62, 81, 85, 123, 147, 160, 163
progestogen-only contraception 11, 53–4
protein 109, 186, 187–8
proximal hamstring tendinopathy (PHT) 118–19
pulmonary embolism 163, 164

relative energy deficiency (REDs) 56, 181–2
relaxation 40–1
resistance training 92, 97
restless leg syndrome (RLS) 31–2
rope skipping 92

running benefits, menopause and 13–15, 65, 96–7, 105, 155–6
  challenges 15–16
  mental health 155–6
  osteoarthritis 98–100
  symptoms 15, 17, 144–5
  see also mindset, positive; nutrition; strength training; training adaptations, menopause; training plans

St John's Wort 174
sarcopenia 107–9
screen time 33
sedentary lifestyle 128–30
sex 18, 51, 166
sexually transmitted infections (STIs) 51
shoulder, frozen 116–17
skin health 132–3, 142, 166
  actinic keratoses 139
  basal cell carcinoma 139–40
  chafing 133–4
  flushing 135–6
  long-term conditions 142
  malignant melanoma 140
  sagging 137
  sensitivities and rashes 136
  sun damage 138–40
  when to see your GP 141, 142
  your feet 137
sleep 18, 40, 111, 124, 130, 146, 151, 154
  causes of poor sleep during menopause 29, 30–2
  importance of good sleep 28, 32
  improving 32–4, 160–1, 172
  treatments 35–6
  when to see your doctor 34
smoking 21, 66, 95
social health and connection 14, 41–2, 154, 155–6
sportswear 61, 63–4, 133–4
sprint interval training (SIT) 202–3
strength training 65, 66, 73, 92, 109, 112, 113, 153, 203, 271–2, 273–374
  barriers to 272
  benefits 271–2
  choosing a weight 174–5
  core work 274
  plyometrics 274
  timing workouts 275–6
  unilateral work 274
  Workout 1: Bodyweight Strength and Plyometrics 285
    A1: double pogo jumps 286
    A2: curtsy lunge to knee drive 287
    B1: reverse lunge to knee drive 288
    B2: skater jumps 289
    C1: squat jumps 290
    C2: single-leg sit to stand 291
    D1: burpees 292
    D2: double lateral hops 293
  Workout 1: Strength 276
    exercises
    A1: squat side walk 277
    A2: narrow squat to high knee 278
    B1: single-leg deadlift 279

B2: single-arm row 280
C1: reverse lunge 281
C2: squat to high pull 282
D1: kneel to push press 283
D2: single-leg glute bridge 284–5
Workout 3: Core 293
A1: inchworm 294
A2: renegade row 295
B1: birddog 296
B2: mountain climbers 297
C1: deadbugs 298
C2: glute bridge 299
D1: side plank leg raise 300
D2: plank 301
stress fractures 93–4
stress levels 17, 45, 45, 111, 123–4, 146, 147–8, 153, 155, 160
sunburn 138–9
supplements and herbal remedies 25, 36, 43, 46, 61, 97, 104, 174–6, 190, 191, 192, 193, 194–5, 196
surgical menopause 7
symptoms, differing experiences of menopause 6, 8, 17–18
symptoms, menopause *see* individual symptoms by name
synovial fluid 100–2, 104

tendon health 115–19
testing hormones 10, 11
testosterone 5, 123, 133, 136, 147
thyroid disorders 11, 43–5, 51, 95, 112
timing of menopause and perimenopause 6–7, 18
tiredness *see* energy levels
training adaptations, menopause
balance and coordination 209–10, 274
cross training 210
dynamic stretches 208
essential
jump and hop/plyometrics 204, 274
making an honest assessment of yourself 198–9
rest and recovery 204–6
run more slowly 201–2
sprint interval training (SIT) 202–3
warm-up and cooling down 199–201, 219
flexibility 207
sample week 211–12
static stretching 207–8
treadmill running 211

training plans 213
adapting your plan 216
fartlek workout 217
half marathon plans
Level 1 214, 220–5
Level 2 214, 226–32
Level 3 214, 232–9
heart rate training zones 218–19
hill repeats workout 218
hill sprints 217–18
how the plans work 215–16
interval runs 218
long runs and easy runs 217
marathon plans
Level 1 215, 240–9
Level 2 215, 250–8
Level 3 215, 258–69
steady runs 217
strides 217
tranexamic acid 53
treatments for HRT, non-HRT
acupuncture 177
CBT 171
clonidine 171
fezolinetant 172
gabapentin 172
herbal treatments 174–5
nutrition 173–4
pregabalin 172
SSRIs and SNRIs 171–2
see also strength training

uterine polyps 50

vaginal bleeding, post-menopause 164
vitamins and minerals 43, 46, 61, 97, 104
calcium 191
iron 43, 189
magnesium 192
vitamin B12 43, 190–1
vitamin C 189
vitamin D 97, 104, 190
vitamin E 61
VO2 max 42, 202
vulva irritation 17

warm-ups and cool-downs 102, 199–201, 219
weight issues 14, 18, 46, 51, 96, 103, 115, 120–31, 179–80, 197

yoga 97, 273